Contract For A Healthy Life

Teens Taking Charge of Their Health

A Guide for Teachers

Cathleen Hamill

authorHOUSE®

AuthorHouse™
1663 Liberty Drive
Bloomington, IN 47403
www.authorhouse.com
Phone: 1 (800) 839-8640

Published by AuthorHouse 07/07/2017

ISBN: 978-1-4208-3721-6 (sc)

CONTRACT FOR A HEALTHY LIFE
STUDENT RESPONSES

"I finally feel like I know what is going on when I go to class!"... Peter

"This is a program I can use forever, it really works!"....
Heather

"I needed something to get me moving and I found it"...
Karl

"When I walk down the hall I notice that kids treat me better, that's because I learned to treat me better"...
Catherine

"I'll use this a lot when I get to high school and go through so many changes, I'll know how to adjust."...
Kim

"This helped me a lot and my parents like the changes too"...
Alex

"I really learned how to help myself"...
Tim

"I feel that my self-esteem has also improved a great deal. I feel better about myself and now know that this project helped me understand that I can accomplish improvements in myself. If I need to change something about myself, I have the ability to do it" . . .
Dennis

Table of Contents

ACKNOWLEDGEMENTS

The years I have spent learning to be a health teacher have been enormously gratifying. I have met many interesting people in the health and teaching professions who have been a tremendous resource for information, clarification, and encouragement in writing this program. I am extremely grateful to those who have helped me to understand how to balance my life and to make a difference in the lives of our students. I want to personally thank each of you for your support and for keeping me accountable to sustain many positive changes in and out of the classroom.

Tina Bengermino ~ without your friendship, wisdom, and energy this could never have been completed.

Dr. Jerry Ainsworth ~ your ideas are inspiring. They are the seedlings for this work.

Reverend Stuart Brush, your definition of spiritual health contributed to developing a deeper meaning for our classroom definition of spiritual health.

Tina Bengermino, Sharon Kowalchick, Pat Lowell, Patty Eng ~ Thanks to each of you for activating this project in each of your own schools and classrooms. This effort provided a great source of confidence and encouragement.

Fairfield Woods Middle School Administration and Health Curriculum Coordinator Lori Mediate, thank you for your encouragement and support.

My children, Sean, Jamie, Michael, and Kevin, thank you for helping me learn the many life lessons that support the ideas for this program.

PREFACE

The quality of life is always improved with optimal health; we want to feel and perform the very best we can. Maintaining this sense of well-being can be difficult as we journey through the challenges of life experiences and ultimately we need to re-evaluate and adjust behaviors that will manage and improve our overall health. This program offers opportunity for students to identify personal health behaviors and initiate improvement in the way they feel and perform physically, mentally, and spiritually.

When I first began teaching sixth, seven, and eighth grade students, I researched and found myself poring over health curriculum books. While sifting through lessons and teaching strategies, I began teaching "by the book." and later discovered I wanted to reach "outside of the box." I wanted more hands-on activities for better application of the information I learned during my graduate studies. I did not want my students simply to listen to me, but to take an active role in their learning. Together we began discussing the meaning of health. I had them write their definition of health in a journal. We discovered that few of us had the same definition or vision of what health meant. We decided that before we could learn about health-related topics, we needed to identify a common definition of health that we could reference when needed. During class discussion we identified three components we agreed should be included in our definition of health. These components are physical, mental, and spiritual health. We shared strategies that are already in place to help maintain, improve, and manage physical, mental, and spiritual wellbeing. For example, consulting a doctor for physical health, reaching out for counseling or religious guidance for spiritual health, or reviewing facts with a teacher for mental health. These resources are extremely valuable and seeking expert information is always encouraged. This program encourages self-reflection and offers strategies that promote self-advocacy in taking care of your own health.

The many demands and challenges we face daily can make the goal of optimal health difficult to achieve. Our most important resource for managing these challenges is education. Education and greater awareness take an active role in supporting personal well-being. We want students to understand and explore ways to embrace both traditional and holistic methods of healthy living. Contract for a Healthy Life is an educational tool that supplements an individual's quest for optimal well-being. Students examine how practicing a healthy lifestyle presently promotes a brighter future. They will feel empowered as they create a vital and fulfilling lifestyle while adjusting daily health patterns. This comprehensive guide on health, wellness, and behavior modification can put knowledge into action. Students have made a difference in the way they feel and perform physically, spiritually, and mentally. Contract for a Healthy Life offers strategies that encourage healthy behaviors and foster a balanced and healthy lifestyle. If you are ready to empower yourself and your students, let us begin the journey and make a positive impact on the future.

INTRODUCTION

I was a student at Southern Connecticut State College graduate school when Dr. Jerry Ainsworth introduced our class to the "12 ingredients of Health." In his upcoming book _Love and Health_, he identifies four daily behaviors: food, rest, exercise, and elimination that help balance and maintain physical, mental, and spiritual health. I introduced this concept into my eighth grade health classes and combined it with our class definition of physical, mental, and spiritual health. I designed a health questionnaire for students to score their personal health behaviors and these results are applied to two "personal health graphs". Students then implement strategies to improve their health using a 6- 8-week behavior modification contract designed to meet personal goals. The program also addresses National and State Health Curriculum standards and objectives. The title of this program is Contract for a Healthy Life. Students commit to changing one aspect of their health using strategies that enable them to manage, improve, reduce, or increase a lifestyle behavior. They make changes that help improve self-awareness, self-esteem, and physical and mental abilities. Assessment rubrics evaluate the final verbal and visual student presentations. I often find students are extremely pleased with their efforts to improve their health. Here is one example.

Our classroom goal for the first few days is to define health and identify behaviors that improve or impair health. After completing our health definition, students take the survey that reflects personal health and then explore strategies to improve one part of their health. Here is Jakes story:

Jake, an eighth grade student came to class the first week looking and acting very tired. Jake seemed too tired to participate in class discussions or activities. After class one day, I asked him why he seemed so tired and he shared that he usually goes to bed between 12:00 and 1:00 a.m. every night. After discussing his nighttime routine and its effects, I suggested he use the health contract to improve his physical rest. We discussed some possible benefits if he increased his sleep. Reluctantly, he bought into the idea of using a contract and designed a "measurement tool" that recorded his progress and encouraged him to gradually change his bedtime from 1:00 a.m. back to 10:30 p.m. Initially Jake found it difficult to eliminate some unhealthy habits, like watching a popular television show until midnight and staying on the computer for great lengths of time. Eventually he began changing his schedule. One day we were beginning a new health topic and I asked questions of the class. To my surprise, Jake raised his hand to answer several of the questions. I checked in with him at times asking him about his progress to improve his sleep and he said he was working on it. At the end of 8 weeks, Jake gave his presentation to the class and shared his progress. Not only did he improve his sleep pattern, he felt more alert and able to concentrate during class lessons. Jake found that his teachers were pleased with his increased participation in class. Their encouragement motivated him to improve his study habits and complete more homework assignments. As his success in school improved, Jake noticed that his relationship with his parents also improved. His parents were pleased with his new study habits and he noticed the stress level in the house decreased. This contract improved Jake's mental performance in school and his relationships at home. He felt better about himself and made a dramatic change in his daily living by changing his sleep pattern. Jake's goal was to change one behavior; to increase his number of hours of sleep. He discovered that this adjustment improved his physical health and greatly improved his mental and spiritual health. The purpose of Contract for a Healthy Life is to enable students to experience this same kind of success. They can examine their physical, mental, and spiritual health and identify areas that need improvement.

It is difficult for anyone to remain completely balanced physically, mentally, and spiritually. Life experiences and events can change the way one feels from day to day. Tracing the roots of unbalanced health and then implementing adjustments can make a difference in the way you feel every day. With the information in this guide, you and your students can identify and adjust a weak area of health, choose a support person, create a measuring tool to record progress, and improve overall health. Your class will discover that when one part of health is balanced, it can positively affect other areas of health as well.

Let us begin with the foundations that will help you create a health program that works for you and your students. Included in this guide are the three areas of health and their definitions:

Physical: *any biological function related to the systems of the body*

Mental: *your ability to reason* (identify, define, calculate, evaluate)

Spiritual: *how you feel about yourself and interact with the world around you using the greater values of humankind.*

I will go into further detail about these components later. Each of these components requires daily attention to maintain a healthy balance. The four daily requirements that nurture a healthy balance are food, rest, exercise, and elimination in each component of health. So, for example, not only is it necessary to feed the physical body with a variety of foods, one must feed information to the brain for mental efficiency and love to the heart and soul for spiritual well-being. The daily requirements for rest, exercise, and elimination apply to physical, mental and spiritual health and these four daily requirements combined with each of the three areas of health are "the 12 ingredients of health". Students explore health improvement strategies offered in Contract for a Healthy Life and learn to balance physical, mental, and spiritual health while practicing the four daily requirements. Your students will learn to identify the area of health that requires improvement for better health and engage in behavior strategies needed to experience a higher level of well-being.

This guide is part of the eighth grade health curriculum. The following page includes health-related curriculum topics that identify units of study teachers can adapt for a behavior improvement program. Also included are strategies that modify the program for a variety of other educational or personal objectives. Inner-city social workers have implemented modifications for individual students having trouble both in and out of school. Contract for a Healthy Life is flexible so that individuals, groups, or families can identify goals that facilitate improvement individually or as a group. Over the years, students consistently demonstrate how powerful Contract for a Healthy Life is as each makes a difference in their daily life. Practicing behaviors that promote optimal health will make you look, feel, and perform better in all areas of your life.

Health Related Topics

PHYSICAL

UNIVERSAL PRECAUTIONS

EXERCISE   RISK FACTORS

EATING DISORDERS

SUBSTANCE USE AND ABUSE

NUTRITION   STRESS

DISEASE PREVENTION

DIVERSITY

HYGIENE

SUICIDE PREVENTION

ADDICTION

SUPPORT SYSTEMS   BODY IMAGE

DECISION-MAKING

DEFINITION OF HEALTH   RELATIONSHIPS – SOCIAL SKILLS

ASSESSMENT OF HEALTH   CONFLICT RESOLUTION

COMMUNICATION   STRESS MANAGEMENT

CONFLICT RESOLUTION   VIOLENCE PREVENTION

PROBLEM SOLVING   GRIEF MANAGEMENT

SELF-ESTEEM

MENTAL   # SPIRITUAL

DEFINING PHYSICAL, MENTAL, AND SPIRITUAL HEALTH

He who has Health has hope; and he who has hope has everything.

~ Arabian Proverb

DEFINING HEALTH: THE BALANCE

If the three areas of health - physical, mental, and spiritual, - were in a perfectly balanced pie graph, it would look like this:

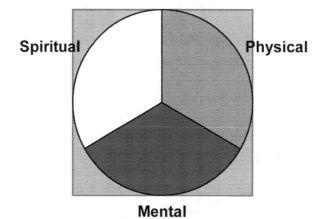

Maintaining perfect balance is difficult, especially when faced with unforeseen life events such as illness, accidents, or a failed personal relationship. The key to happiness is to practice behaviors that improve and balance our physical, mental and spiritual health. We feel our best when we are content and healthy in all areas of our health. For better understanding, we will begin with a complete definition of physical, mental, and spiritual health and identify the behaviors required to maintain a healthy balance. We will also compare healthy and unhealthy behaviors identified as high and low-quality behaviors that affect a healthy balance. Finally, we will compare the effects each area of health has on the other two.

PHYSICAL HEALTH

To keep the body in good health is a duty…otherwise, we shall not be able to keep our mind strong and clear.
~ Buddha

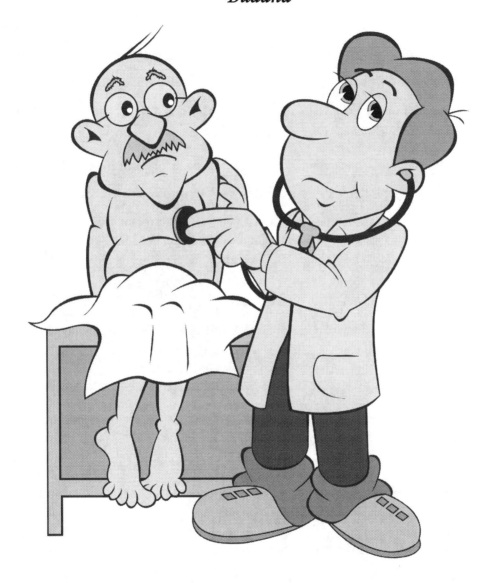

"If your muscles were as hard as your arteries,
you would be in great shape."

PHYSICAL HEALTH

ANY BIOLOGICAL FUNCTION RELATED TO THE SYSTEMS OF THE BODY

Our bodies are miraculous machines with systems that function together to maintain good health and protect us from harm. Below is a list of the thirteen body systems. Students learn how systems support one another. For example, the skeletal system has to work in harmony with the muscular system or neither of them will function properly. Keeping both systems strong and healthy can ensure each will function at its best. The immune system relies on the circulatory system to help deliver needed antibodies for protection from disease. Both must function properly for the whole body to benefit. The 13 systems include:

1.	Digestive	7.	Nervous
2.	Circulatory	8.	Reproductive
3.	Muscular	9.	Respiratory
4.	Skeletal	10.	Integumentary
5.	Cardiovascular	11.	Excretory
6.	Endocrine	12.	Urinary
		13.	Immune

When each system is functioning optimally, we feel our best. When one system is not one hundred percent efficient, its shortfall can compromise the balance of health as a whole. Practicing high-quality behaviors encourages improved efficiency. For example, nutrition plays an important role in nurturing the organs, tissues, and cells that work together to keep us healthy. What you eat can determine how you feel, look, and behave. Practicing a healthy diet is a high-quality behavior. A low quality diet can lead to weight gain, fatigue, anxiety, headaches and a suppressed immune system. As often occurs, spiritual and mental health can be affected by this behavior as well. While practicing a poor diet, a person might feel depressed because he/she is gaining weight. He/she might not concentrate as effectively because he/she is consuming too much caffeine or sugar. In this instance, a poor diet has compromised physical, spiritual and mental well-being. A person with an unhealthy diet might have a health graph that looks like this:

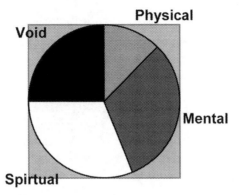

Without corrective strategies, this imbalance may negatively affect the physical, mental, and spiritual well-being for many years. As we explore the need for optimal physical health, students learn how healthy choices make a difference in their daily life. Students may choose to improve their rest, diet, or exercise. They may increase water intake, fruits or vegetables, flossing, or brushing their teeth. Some reduce sugar or fat intake. Improving physical health helps maintain and manage the synchronization needed for all the body systems to function proficiently.

MENTAL HEALTH

Knowledge is love, light, and vision...
~ Helen Keller

MENTAL HEALTH:
THE ABILITY TO REASON

Ask a group of people for their definition of mental health and the answer and interpretation may vary dramatically. When I ask my students for this definition, most often they combine it with their interpretation of emotional and social health. They understand that mental health is part of the brain. For better clarification, we take time to differentiate the characteristics between mental and emotional health. To begin, I use an example about my young dog, Ernie. First, I ask my students how they would respond if I told them that 2+2=5. They always try to correct me and then I insist that I was wrong and actually 2+2=3. Frustrated, they give me the correct answer: 2+2=4. I then ask them how they think my favorite puppy, Ernie, would respond if I told him that 2+2=5. We all agree that Ernie would be his usual playful self, but he would not understand or care that the equation is incorrect. We talk about the ability humans have to reason. Most of us have the ability to reason that 2+2=4, but Ernie's' ability to reason is not as great. He can use reasoning to solve some problems, like when he was so thirsty in the summer; he found the birdbath to get a drink of water. We thought he was a genius! However, Ernie's ability to reason is limited.

The human ability to reason enables us to decipher, compare, evaluate, contrast, calculate, define, identify, and make informed decisions. Emotions are not necessary for us to do this. Our mental health combines intellect and memory to make useful determinations. There are different levels of mental capabilities that are determined by heredity, academic behaviors, illness, and quality of information. A low I.Q., poor study habits, or inadequate education can contribute to limited mental performance. Our mental health diminishes when memory and making decisions are impaired due to drug abuse, mental illness, or age.

Our mental health is just as important to us as our physical and spiritual health. Exercising high-quality behaviors such as applying knowledge, reading, writing, and listening enables us to maintain and improve our mental performance. Our ability to think fosters new ideas and deeper insight.

These exercises, combined with greater knowledge, can stimulate and inspire creativity, innovation, and curiosity.

Mental health does not require feelings or social attachments in order to function properly; however, our spiritual and physical health can definitely affect how well we function mentally. If someone is depressed or angry, these emotions can interfere with concentration and judgment. Physical fatigue can interrupt one's ability to remember information. Other low-quality behaviors that interfere with mental health and the ability to reason or create include retaining incorrect information, disorganized study habits, and poor listening skills. Practicing high-quality behaviors that enhance our creativity and the ability to reason helps to balance our health as a whole.

A person whose mental health is diminished may have a health graph that looks like this:

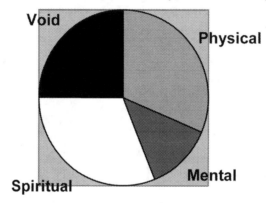

Once again, one area of health can directly affect another.

Students who choose to improve their mental health may increase their reading or studying, correct incorrect answers on tests, quizzes, and essays, or reorganize study materials. When students select this area of health to work on, they will improve academic performance in school.

Let us examine our third area of health, Spiritual Health.

SPIRITUAL HEALTH

*What lies behind us and what lies before us are small
matters compared to what lies within us...
~ Ralph Waldo Emerson*

SPIRITUAL HEALTH:

HOW YOU FEEL ABOUT YOURSELF AND INTERACT WITH THE WORLD AROUND YOU USING THE GREATER VALUES OF HUMANKIND

For many people spiritual health is the most important part of their life. When I first started teaching health, I did not use the title *spiritual health* as part of my health definition. It was a word some educators felt uncomfortable using because for many its meaning has a close connection to religion. With so many different religions and opinions about religion, it seemed risky to offer this as part of my definition of health. Many health educators refer to this part of health as the emotional or social component. Some teachers even use both titles as part of the definition of health. I decided to explore the meaning of this health component. I found that emotional health emphasized how feelings and emotions like anger, sadness, elation, etc., are managed, but it did not encompass other elements I found important. Social health focused on interaction with others but this too lacked clarity for this area of health. Using spiritual health as part of the whole definition of health was the best fit for my interpretation.

I use the title *spiritual* health because its definition includes components such as emotional health and social interaction, as well as self-esteem, self-worth, serenity, values, and conflict resolution. I also discovered that I felt comfortable introducing religion in proper context with my curriculum.

The foundation of spiritual health begins in infancy and is the core of our self-worth. The amount of love, attention, comfort, and direction contributed by our family and their response to our accomplishments or failures establishes self-worth. Do we feel successful with our efforts? Do we receive encouragement that motivates us to continue to be productive? These external factors influence our internal spiritual health. We develop a sense of self and as we grow, accumulate values as part of a system that is reliable for decision-making. Positive role modeling teaches healthy values that are important in a family. Honesty, trust, and integrity are some of the greater values of humankind. We may begin to understand and practice these values when challenged with difficult decisions. These practices are high-quality behaviors. When defining the greater values of humankind within our definition of spiritual health, students understand better when I share a story that happened in our family years ago when my four children were very young.

It was during the summer when two of their friends were staying with us for the week and we decided to take the ferry over to Long Island for shopping, lunch, and ice cream. Each child had a small allowance for the day and we had a great time. On the way home, my son, Michael, spotted a truck with a flat tire at the side of the exit ramp. He saw a man standing on the side of the van and said to me "Mom, we have to help that man". My initial response was that the man was a stranger and it wasn't safe to stop, but once all the kids reminded me that we had always taught them to offer help to others in need, I decided to pull over and ask if he needed help. He said he was on his way home when the tire went flat and then discovered he did not have a spare tire. I offered to take him to the local gas station to find a tire. The gas station attendant said he only had a few tires and did not know if any of them would fit the rim of the van. He suggested we go to the next town where there was a tire store. When we got to the store, we discovered that it had just closed. We went back to the gas station and the attendant said to bring the tire rim to him so that he could fit the tire. On our way back to get the rim, my son, Kevin, noticed a homeless man at the bottom of the exit ramp with a sign asking for money or food. Kevin looked at me and said, "Mom we have to help that man". I smiled and asked him what he thought we should do. As we waited for the first man to get the tire rim from his van, the six kids collected all of their left over change from the day. They gathered almost $12.00 and asked me to deliver it to the homeless man. As I walked back to give him their money, the other man came back to the car with the tire rim and unbeknownst to me gave each of the children money for ice cream. We drove back to the gas station and waited for the tire to be mounted on the rim. We struck up a conversation and the man shared his story with us. He came to the United States two years earlier with little money and his large family. They were from Haiti and he traveled two hours each way to work every day to help make ends meet. It seemed a difficult but satisfying life for him and we all enjoyed the reflection. We exchanged other stories from our past and then took the repaired tire back to his van. It was getting late and we wished each other well and said our good-byes. As he walked back up the exit ramp to his van, I noticed the children with money in their hands and they told me he insisted they take it. We talked about his story and the reason we stopped and decided that we should give the money back to him for his children. I walked up the side of the ramp, talked to the man for a few more minutes, and gave him back the money. As I walked to my car, the homeless man passed me and mentioned that he wanted to help change the tire on the van. I continued and a different man began walking up the ramp carrying two bags of fast food and I was curious. I asked him where he was going. He said he lived across the street and sat on his porch every afternoon. He saw the events of our long afternoon unfold and decided to go to the nearest fast food restaurant to pick up food for each of the men.

As we drove home, we talked about the adventures of our day. We talked about the ferry ride, things we bought at the stores, and the food we ate. In the end, we all agreed that the best part of the day was when we stopped to help someone and the gesture became infectious. Everyone involved in the journey felt warm and good inside. When I think of this story I realize that kindness, empathy, trust, and thoughtfulness was a big part of our day. The decision to practice these values made a difference for each of us and for people we had never met before. The small gesture to help another person in need motivated others to want to do the same. This one journey together raised self-esteem and had a direct effect on everyone's day. I enjoy sharing this story with my students. It is a great example of the power of the greater values of humankind and its connection to spiritual health.

As we develop our value system, daily events and challenges can encourage us to use high-quality behaviors and make healthy decisions. The more frequently we exercise healthy choices, the better equipped we are to do the same when facing high-risk situations. If we practice high-quality behaviors to exercise our spiritual health, we develop a strong sense of self-worth that makes us feel good about ourselves. Self-worth influences an internal barometer that regulates our level of confidence. This is what we call self-esteem.

Self-esteem is the degree of confidence we demonstrate through our behaviors and establishes how comfortable we are with ourselves, others, and change. Esteem has a direct effect on our happiness, sense of humor, and the way we interact in the world. This internal barometer formulates interpretations and perspectives about life and affects our behavior responses. The greater our self esteem is, the more we can respond confidently to change, criticism, reflection, tolerance, and differences in others. For example, when others analyze specific behaviors or offer advice, how do I respond? Do I have an open mind or do I shut down and ignore the possibility that I may need to make changes?

As we grow older, a style of conflict resolution evolves using passive, assertive, or aggressive coping strategies that affect our emotions and overall health. Emotions are symptoms of self-esteem and can greatly affect our relationships with others. Emotions are the result of any experience that affects self-esteem. Self-esteem influences happiness and the way we respond to success and failure.

In the pursuit of happiness, one will have both positive and negative life experiences. The way we manage our life experiences is an essential part of spiritual health. Life events are our greatest teachers and often affect our outlook. We are students who learn from accomplishments and failures and sometimes we learn more in the darkness than in the light. Adversity greatly affects spiritual health, especially because these experiences are opportunities that enable us to learn and grow most.

I believe there is another and even deeper sense of contentment that we pursue which is as important as happiness: *serenity*. Serenity is an inner peace that allows us to manage emotions with a belief that we can accept any life experience with grace because there are events we cannot control. Serenity enables us to move through transitions gracefully even when confronted with failures, hardships, and other life changes. We learn to accept things we cannot control as normal. A well-developed sense of serenity fosters an inner peace that is greater than emotions such as happiness. As serenity is nourished, it helps direct us to a fuller spiritual sense of well-being. I have met numerous elderly people who continue to thrive as they maneuver through the challenges of getting older. Amongst them are a few who have lost their soul mate but still carry an aura of serenity. They demonstrate a presence of grace as they accept things they cannot control.

Practicing high-quality behaviors that encourage a strong sense of self-worth, self-esteem and serenity enhance spiritual health and enable us to manage life experiences in a healthy way. Behaviors such as caring for others, practicing forgiveness and compassion, and demonstrating empathy, help foster a strong sense of spiritual health. These practices can have a direct effect on maturity and developmental growth. The characteristics of spiritual health help cultivate a balanced alignment between healthy attitude and healthy behaviors. If a solid foundation has been established using high-quality behaviors, every experience will offer the opportunity to choose a positive path.

Students who chose to improve their spiritual health as part of their health project may choose to increase caring for others, enhance family relationships, improve anger management, and find ways to raise self-esteem.

THE FOUR DAILY REQUIREMENTS

FOOD, REST, EXERCISE, AND ELIMINATION

BEHAVIORS THAT PROMOTE BALANCE:

FOOD, REST, EXERCISE, ELIMINATION

The journey between what you once were and who you are now becoming is where the dance of life really takes place...
~ Barbara De Angelis

We have defined three components of health: physical, mental and spiritual health. Each of these components help maintain a healthy balance when nurtured with the four daily requirements; food, rest, exercise, and elimination. We will now identify these requirements and provide examples for each. Students will then select one improvement and create a behavior modification strategy to improve their health over an 8-week period.

Taking time to identify high and low-quality choices that fuel, rest, exercise, and eliminate physical, mental, and spiritual health is important as we continue to finalize our complete definition of health. Now, let us examine the behaviors that promote a healthy balance physically, mentally, and spiritually. The required daily behaviors essential for optimal health include food, rest, exercise, and elimination in all three areas of our health. This means that it is necessary to fuel, rest, exercise, and eliminate physically, mentally, and spiritually each day. The objective is to satisfy the requirements with high-quality choices and behaviors that promote good health. It is important to identify how high-quality and low-quality choices influence the balance of health. Better understanding about these choices enables students to develop critical thinking when making decisions regarding their health contracts.

We begin this process as we examine examples of food, rest, exercise, and elimination and their effect on physical health. This same exercise will then identify behaviors and choices that affect mental and spiritual health. During class discussion, I draw a large illustration of the health pie graph divided into three equal parts, each representing one of the three components of health. Numbers one through four are in each section and we begin to define and identify the four daily requirements: 1. food, 2. rest, 3. exercise, and 4. elimination, as they apply to physical, mental, and spiritual health. For example, students share favorite foods as they identify high-quality or low-quality choices for physical food. One student may select an apple and another, a candy bar, as choices for physical food and I list them on the pie graph under the section for physical food. One choice identified as high quality, the other low quality and during class discussion, students decide how high and low-quality choices affect physical health, long and short-term. Students use this same process to identify choices for rest, exercise and elimination in all three areas of health.

Within the pie graph, we identify choices for mental health. High-quality knowledge improved because of reading or listening. These are examples of mental food and mental exercise. Knowledge is mental food and reading is mental exercise. The higher quality the food, the more effective is the ability to reason. Those who avoid reading or listening to others limit their mental exercise and therefore minimize mental efficiency.

Following is a brief description identifying each of the 4 daily requirements as they apply to each component of health. The result of physical, mental, and spiritual health fortified daily with food, rest, exercise, and elimination is called "the 12 ingredients of health".

PHYSICAL FOOD

Don't dig your grave with your knife and fork...
~ English Proverb

As we explore examples of physical foods, often students will respond with foods such as apples or pizza. These foods contribute to fueling the body for energy and we identify these as high-quality foods because of their nutritional value. For some students, their favorite food is chocolate candy, and this is identified as a low-quality food because it does not offer important nutrients needed for optimal physical performance. Whether you choose a high-quality or low-quality food, when any food is ingested, the body has been fueled. When choices for food are consistently high- quality foods, our body will perform more efficiently for a longer period of time. During class I offer an analogy as an example that demonstrates how high and low-quality choices make a difference. When choosing between high-quality and low-quality octane gasoline for cars, the better gasoline will ensure better car performance for a longer period of time. When choices for physical food are consistently low-quality, we experience a future with too much fat, high cholesterol and high blood pressure. These problems can be long-term and affect an individual's lifetime well-being. The U.S. Department of Agriculture has suggested using the Food Guide Pyramid as a reference for a healthy diet. This food chart is one resource student's use to record progress while improving their diet as part of their Contract for a Healthy Life.

PHYSICAL REST

Most students respond with sleep as the best form of physical rest. If their hours of sleep is within the recommended number of hours needed for optimal health, this is considered high-quality rest. The National Children's Organization recommends 91/2 hours of sleep per night for middle school children. (Reference)I have discovered that many students don't get the recommended number hours of sleep or their sleep is often interrupted. This is defined as low-quality rest. It's interesting to note that many students overlook the value of healthy sleep and its importance on academic performance as well as social interaction with others. During this project, students who choose to readjust their sleep patterns and improve their sleep eventually notice the positive results this change has on academic performance and personal relationships. A low-quality behavior such as poor sleep contributes to poor concentration and affects mental performance. Fatigue also contributes to difficulty getting along with others. Physical rest affects all areas of our health and is important for optimal performance in each. While implementing strategies to increase their sleep, students are practicing a high-quality behavior that can affect their daily life in a positive way. Improved general well-being, better grades and study skills, and improved interaction with others are some of the findings students are pleased with as they share their final project with the class.

PHYSICAL EXERCISE

No longer conscious of my movement, I discovered a new unity with nature. I had found a new source of power and beauty; a source I never dreamed existed....

~ Roger Bannister (first person to break the four-minute mile)

Physical exercises are easy for students to identify. Most of them are involved in some form of physical exercise simply because of their age. For the most part, they seem to enjoy physical exercise and often this is the strongest area of their health. Swimming, biking, playing soccer, and dancing are common activities at this age. These are considered high-quality exercises and help to improve performance in many of the body systems. To demonstrate the importance of physical exercise, I sometimes use an example of a broken bone that is immobilized in a cast for several weeks. The bone must be still for a lengthy time in order for it to heal and realign itself. In this instance, even though the surrounding muscles are not injured, they must be immobilized to allow the bone to heal. When the cast is removed, the function of the limb or area that has been injured is temporarily compromised until the surrounding atrophied muscles are rehabilitated. When therapists manipulate and exercise muscles for paralysis patients, their purpose is to reduce atrophy in the muscles that cannot move.

Any muscle that does not exercise for long periods of time will experience atrophy and diminished physical performance. All muscles, including the heart, can be affected this way. Consistent high-quality exercises help keep the body physically strong and fit. There are some activities such as bowling, golf, or croquet that offer some physical exercise. These activities are valued more for their social benefits and may be considered low quality physical exercises. A lifestyle that engages in a variety of exercises benefits all of the body systems and promotes a healthy balance. Students who want to improve their physical exercise may strive to improve timed running distances or increase physical activity each week. Some students design a schedule for weight lifting and weekly exercise classes.

PHYSICAL ELIMINATION

When I ask students for examples of physical elimination, their first response is almost always related to urination or bowel movements. We then talk about what is considered physical waste and reasons they are eliminated. We explore other examples of waste, such as dead cells, bacteria, viruses, mucous, germs, and carbon dioxide. Even baby teeth are eventually considered a physical waste. Students discover the importance of elimination as it relates to discomfort, illness, or even death. Each system of the body provides a means for eliminating waste. The body eliminates the wastes using physical functions such as coughing, sneezing, vomiting, peeling, perspiring, bleeding, exhaling etc. Elimination is beneficial because it helps to keep the body clean and free from harmful agents that may cause illness. We sometimes facilitate elimination by brushing our teeth, flossing, showering, clipping our nails, or cutting our hair. It's fascinating to explore the many ways the body eliminates wastes. Other high-quality behaviors that facilitate elimination include healthful dieting, washing our hands, blowing our nose, cleaning our ears, etc. An example of low-quality elimination is labored breathing and exhaling due to asthma or emphysema. Elimination is a form of prevention and maintenance that promotes good health. Students who choose to improve physical elimination may follow a healthy diet and record weight loss. Some students record the number of times they floss either daily or weekly. Students sometimes increase their daily fluid intake and compare number of seasonal illnesses.

MENTAL FOOD

The brain is where mental health is centered. This organ requires fuel or food to function optimally. Information and knowledge are considered food for the brain and when fed with high-quality information and knowledge, mental health is improved. The greater amount of high-quality information, the more effectively the brain performs academically. Greater knowledge enhances skills for decision making, creativity, evaluating, comparing and contrasting, identifying, and defining. There are some mental foods that are regarded as better quality food. High-quality mental foods include academic information, facts, quality television programs, and informative presentations. Examples of low-quality foods are cartoons, comic strips, gossip, lies. These resources offer minimal information without benefits for more meaningful knowledge. Students who want to improve mental food may choose to increase their amount of reading. Some students have accumulated and defined new vocabulary words. Others increase study time. Each student who has selected to improve their mental food has successfully improved one or more of their academic grades.

MENTAL REST

Poorly managed mental exercise can result in overwhelming levels of stress or "mental burnout". The "workaholic" is one such example of potential "mental burnout." The need to rest the mind is as important as resting the body. Some people try to rest the mind while abusing drugs, alcohol, or food. These low-quality behaviors are examples of unhealthy choices that lead to serious health risks.

Healthy choices that reduce stress often result in greater amounts of energy and motivation. Strategies to accommodate mental rest include meditation, journaling, listening to music, periodic vacations, and physical exercise. As students commit to practicing these strategies, their recorded discoveries demonstrate how mental rest helps lower stress levels. Many students have acknowledged an improvement in their overall well-being. Interpersonal relationships are improved with lower levels of stress. A student who improves mental rest may record discoveries using a list or chart that monitors stress-related behaviors and responses. Other examples of high-quality mental rest include walks, hobbies, and recreational activities.

MENTAL EXERCISE
The roots of education are bitter, but the fruit is sweet... ~ Aristotle

Identifying mental exercises that improve our mental health is more difficult than identifying physical exercises that improve our physical health. Actually, the thought process that helps us identify these exercises is an example of mental exercise. Identifying, comparing, and evaluating those mental exercises that are high-quality is an example of exercising mentally. Mental exercise improves individual understanding, increases knowledge, encourages creativity and fosters meaningful insight. With high-quality information, increased or improved mental exercise enables greater mental performance and for students, often results in better grades. Examples of mental exercise include reading, writing, solving math problems and completing homework. Many students improve grades while practicing mental exercises that increase study time, correct quizzes, tests, and written assignments, and improve study strategies for homework assignments. Students discuss and compare the effects of playing video games or watching cartoons for long periods of time and how these behaviors minimize the ability to exercise the mind. These are considered low-quality exercises.

MENTAL ELIMINATION

How is it possible to eliminate mentally? It is easier to understand how we eliminate mentally if what we want to eliminate is identified first. Mental waste includes incorrect or useless information. Incorrect test answers, poor spelling and even idle gossip are examples of mental waste. Our brains are equipped to eliminate most incorrect information automatically. Here is an example. I told my students that 2+2=5 and they were able to reason that the answer was incorrect and not useful. They eliminated the equation from their pool of information. If all information is retained without eliminating incorrect information, mental operations would cease to work effectively. Previously, mental health was defined as our ability to reason and my students and I were able to demonstrate reasoning using the three different equations: 2+2=5, 2+2=3 and 2+2=4. We calculated the information and identified the correct answer. The ability to replace incorrect answers with the correct answer demonstrates the value of eliminating useless information so that it does not interfere with the ability to exercise useful information. The elimination process is improved when students facilitate high-quality behaviors such as correcting wrong answers on tests and quizzes, reviewing essays with a teacher, and asking questions for academic clarification. These strategies help to eliminate mental waste and improve mental performance. Many students who design strategies to improve mental elimination apply this process as part of their health contract and successfully achieve higher academic scores.

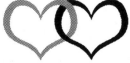

SPIRITUAL FOOD

*Those who bring sunshine to the lives of others cannot
keep it from themselves... James M. Barrie*

The definition of spiritual health establishes the importance of self-worth, self-esteem, and serenity. These elements are nurtured with spiritual foods such as love, encouragement, compliments, and a sense of accomplishment. If you compare the child who receives these spiritual foods abundantly with that of an abused or neglected child, you can better understand how high-quality spiritual food fosters a greater sense of spiritual well-being. An individual will experience greater self-worth and serenity as well as higher self-esteem when spiritual food is part of his or her daily diet. During the eight week Contract for a Healthy Life project, students who seek to increase or improve spiritual food may choose to record and compare affectionate greetings and compliments. They may list acts of encouragement, attention, or acknowledgment from friends and family members. They then record daily discoveries and personal effects. These students discover that greater amounts of spiritual food increase self-esteem and confidence. They also learn how verbal abuse and minimal amounts of attention are examples of low-quality spiritual food and can result in depression, guilt, hatred, bitterness, intolerance and resentment; all examples of spiritual waste.

SPIRITUAL REST
*Let the harm of the year go with it...
~ Molly McCarthy (my grandmother)*

Have you ever known someone who continually cares <u>for</u> others but finds it uncomfortable receiving care <u>from</u> others? This is often someone who needs spiritual rest the most. Taking time to rest spiritually enriches our spiritual health. Spiritual rest helps restore energy, motivation, and a greater sense of well-being. There are many ways to practice spiritual rest with high-quality behaviors. Some examples are quiet reflection, prayer, journaling, self indulgence, and allowing others to care for you. Spiritual rest provides opportunities to regroup emotionally and feel refreshed spiritually. While monitoring behaviors that encourage spiritual rest, students record any physical, mental, or spiritual benefits over an 8 week period of time. Most feel calmer, less stressed, and better prepared for the daily challenges they face.

During class discussion we talk about ways people search for spiritual rest and how this endeavor sometimes leads to poor decisions that result in greater emotional pain. Self-imposed long-term isolation from friends or family members is sometimes perceived as spiritual rest and can lead to harmful side effects such as depression. Many addicts are seeking spiritual rest when they abuse their drug of choice. These behaviors are considered examples of low-quality spiritual rest.

When students choose to improve spiritual rest, they record emotional changes using a daily planner or check-off sheet. They monitor strategies such as listening to music, increasing prayer or quiet time, or embracing behaviors for personal enjoyment. Students who follow this approach often feel empowered as they improve their physical, mental, and spiritual health.

SPIRITUAL EXERCISE
If you do good, people may accuse you of selfish motives. Do good anyway... ~ Mother Teresa

When we do for others we are exercising spiritually. When we do for others without expecting anything in return, we are practicing high-quality spiritual exercise. Spiritual exercise contributes to high self-esteem and a greater sense of self-worth. Caring for another being encourages us to reach beyond our own needs as we search for useful ways to be helpful. This effort embraces a broader sense of purpose and offers the opportunity for reflection and insight. Spiritual exercise encourages positive interaction within interpersonal relationships and community groups. When students choose to increase their spiritual exercise, often they use a measuring tool that lists random acts of kindness. Over time, they will record their discoveries and often these students improve personal relationships and experience greater self-esteem. While many teens rely on outside sources to determine their degree of self-esteem, this is an opportunity for them to discover how they can improve their own self-esteem and confidence. Students find this is a very empowering experience.

During class discussion we also talk about how minimal spiritual exercise impacts spiritual health as much as lack of physical exercise minimizes physical performance. Limited spiritual exercise can result in self-centered individuals who practice self-serving behaviors. Low-quality behaviors that minimize spiritual growth include judging others, practicing prejudice or indifference, manipulating for power or attention, and not taking accountability when hurting others.

SPIRITUAL ELIMINATION

The jealous are troublesome to others but torment to themselves...
~ William Penn

Sometimes people accept and harbor spiritual waste for a long time without realizing it. Concealing spiritual waste can be as harmful as preventing elimination of physical or mental waste. Guilt, stress, hatred, bigotry, envy, jealousy, and bitterness are a few examples of spiritual waste. It is most important to eliminate these wastes to avoid the damaging effects physically, mentally, and spiritually. As students learn the concept of spiritual waste, I use small pieces of paper to demonstrate the burdens these worthless emotions generate. While identifying each piece of paper as examples of hatred, bitterness, or jealousy, I place it on my right or left shoulder. As I accumulate more pieces of paper, I begin to walk laboriously, illustrating how their weight has burdensome effects. During this process we also discuss the value of elimination and cite healthful strategies for removing various spiritual wastes. To finalize the lesson I remove the papers, crumple them up, and throw them in the wastebasket as a symbolic gesture that spiritual waste must be eliminated in order to nurture physical, mental, and spiritual health. Two methods that may initiate elimination include practicing forgiveness and utilizing positive imagery. Other techniques engage in counseling, journaling, or improving communication skills. Identifying the most compatible method for spiritual elimination promotes more opportunities for success.

Students also learn the harmful effects of unhealthy spiritual elimination. Pent up anger, frustration, and disappointment can lead to aggression, abuse or demeaning behaviors. The results can lead to serious consequences and poor health.

OUR HEALTH DEFINES
WHO WE ARE

In the long run we shape our lives and we shape ourselves.
The process never ends until we die. And the choices
we make are ultimately our own responsibility...
~ Eleanor Roosevelt

THE 4 DAILY REQUIREMENTS

1. Apple
2. Sleep
3. Swimming
4. Exhaling CO2

PHYSICAL

1. Academic information
2. Meditation
3. Reading
4. Correcting mistakes

MENTAL

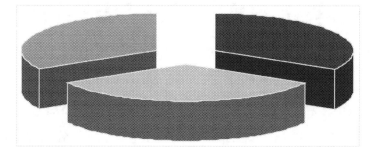

SPIRITUAL

1. Love
2. Allowing others to do for you
3. Helping others
4. Forgive someone

EXAMPLES OF HIGH AND LOW-QUALITY BEHAVIORS

		High Quality	Low Quality
PHYSICAL:			
	1. Food:	apple	candy
	2. Exercise:	swimming	bowling
	3. Rest:	restful sleep	disturbed sleep
	4. Elimination:	exhaling CO2	purging food
MENTAL:			
	1. Food:	academic information	cartoons
	2. Exercise:	reading	doodling
	3. Rest:	meditation	drug use
	4. Elimination:	omitting incorrect information (ex. 2+2=5)	forgetting information
SPIRITUAL:			
	1. Food:	love	co-dependence / neglect
	2. Exercise:	helping others	self-centered actions
	3. Rest:	allowing others to do for you / praying	not allowing others to help you / isolation
	4. Elimination:	forgiveness	aggressive venting, yelling

INTRODUCING TOM AND SALLY

You'll See It When You Believe It: Using Vision

*Look at every situation as if you were in the
future and you were looking back on it...
~ General Peter Schoomaker*

With the information learned about choosing high-quality behaviors that improve our health, a complete definition of optimal health is: <u>Balancing our physical, mental, and spiritual well-being with selected high-quality behaviors to nurture food, rest, exercise, and elimination within each health component.</u>

As new experiences alter our physical, mental, and spiritual health, it is important to adjust behavior patterns that promote optimal health. Sooner or later unhealthy health patterns produce negative outcomes. It's time to practice applying our health knowledge and predict how this could affect our future. I use the following class activity to explore with students the effects of healthy and unhealthy behavior patterns that affect our future.

Let's imagine that we're in high school and two students, Tom and Sally, attend our high school. If each Health Pie Graph is placed next to each other, they might look like this:

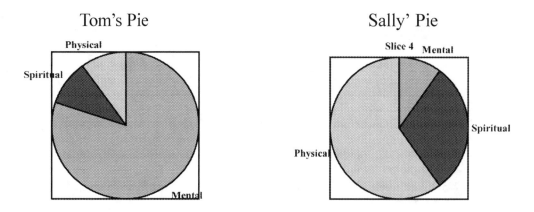

Tom's Pie Graph Sally's Pie Graph

32

As we examine each graph carefully we can learn a lot about each individual. We can actually identify some of their health strengths and weaknesses. Let's examine Tom's health graph.

Tom's graph illustrates that he is very strong mentally but limited physically and spiritually. He is a high school student who has terrific grades. He enjoys reading and using the computer. He actively participates when researching and designing projects. The mental piece of his graph is large because he invests a lot of time nurturing food, rest, exercise, and elimination in this area of his health. But Tom's graph also indicates neglect in his physical and spiritual areas of health. Tom might be a junk food junkie who gets little sleep or exercise because he spends so much time exercising his mental health. He is smart and successful in school and other students recognize this. The time Tom spends on his academic performance affects the quality of his interpersonal relationships. He doesn't socialize much and has few friends. He rarely practices high-quality behaviors that would enhance his spiritual health. Unaware of his imbalance, Tom continues to cultivate his mental health with little regard for his physical and spiritual health.

Sally's strength is in the physical area of health. She gets a lot of exercise because she plays soccer and basketball. She eats a balanced diet and gets lots of rest. Sally practices high-quality behaviors in hygiene and is sick infrequently. She spends much time focusing on her physical health and not enough time on high-quality practices that would enhance her mental performance. Her grades are low and little time is spent reading and reviewing her school assignments. Sally barely gets by academically. But Sally enjoys spending time with her family and friends and often pitches in when they need help. Her spiritual graph indicates that she is presently happy personally and socially.

Both Tom and Sally may be content with the way they live their lives right now. But let's envision their future health if they did not rebalance their health pie graph. We do this activity in class. It's interesting to me that for every academic quarter for the past six years, students always identify Tom and Sally in the same way. Each is always the same person for every class. If Tom and Sally do not readjust their priorities, their life 20 years from now might look like this.

Tom is a commuter who works in a high-powered business company on the top floor of a New York skyscraper. He earns a lot of money and has great responsibility. Tom enjoys his work and spends a great deal of time making his company successful. He lives in a fancy house and drives an expensive car. Tom doesn't eat a well-balanced diet and still prefers junk food. He is 30 pounds overweight, has high cholesterol and blood pressure, and with a heredity factor that indicates a pulmonary weakness, Tom is a heart attack waiting to happen. He did not improve behaviors that would enhance his spiritual health; he is in an unhappy marriage and does not spend much time with his two young children. Tom's health pie graph is still unbalanced. He still spends time maintaining his mental health but has not practiced high-quality behaviors that would improve his physical and spiritual health.

Sally's life 20 years later is quite different from Tom's. She is still physically active and has acquired many friendships over the years. Sally never went to college because her grades were not acceptable. Now Sally teaches aerobics and coaches basketball. She lives in a small apartment and drives an older car. She finds it difficult to make ends meet financially. Sally would like to go back to school but doesn't make the time or money to support an education.

Both Tom and Sally are satisfied with some areas of their lives, but each would like to find a way to improve other areas. Let's take Tom and Sally back to high school, readjust their health pie graphs using high-quality behaviors, and evaluate whether this might make a difference in their futures.

If you were a guidance counselor who had an opportunity to make suggestions for Tom and Sally, what would you advise them to do? For Tom, you might suggest that he join a school activity that would offer opportunities to interact with other students. He could offer tutoring to a peer. He could make more friends, get more involved with community volunteer groups, and improve his spiritual health. Tom could also join a recreational activity or an after-school program for more exercise and social interaction and change to a more balanced diet. Suggestions like these could improve his physical health. These changes might take time away from his mental exercise, but in the long run improve the balance in other areas of his health.

Sally, on the other hand, could benefit with more mental exercise and elimination. A counselor might suggest she take her test and quiz papers back to her teachers and review incorrect information. She could increase her study time by 20-30 minutes each night. Sally could also investigate professional or peer tutoring. These suggestions would help to improve her grades and study habits. Better grades would enable her to apply to college, get a college degree, and place her in a higher financial bracket when applying for future jobs.

For Tom and Sally, rebalancing the physical, mental, and spiritual areas of their health can make a difference in both their present and future lives. If each recognizes the value in these suggestions and practices them regularly, their future lives could be different. Let's examine their futures after adjusting the weaknesses in their health balance.

Tom's social life and friendships improve and he has greater awareness of the needs of others. His new insight enables him to develop relationships in a healthy way and to offer more compatibility in a future family. If Tom changes his physical habits, he could avoid future illness, discomfort, and even a premature death.

Sally's new study habits and academic assistance raise her grades in high school. She improves her vocabulary, and the college of her choice accepts her application. When she graduates, her college education provides greater influence when she applies for a job in a career that interests her. Eventually she can afford to buy a house or condominium and drive a new car.

Tom and Sally are just examples of what an imbalance could predict. There are many people whose lives are similar to Tom's and Sally's. I'm sure each of us knows a Tom or Sally. These examples have illustrated the importance of self-awareness. Implementing strategies to maintain a balance in our physical, mental, and spiritual health can make us look, feel, and perform our best. We have the knowledge and power to strive for our goals and visions using high- quality behaviors that result in a better lifestyle.

Activity: Tom's Pie

Step One:

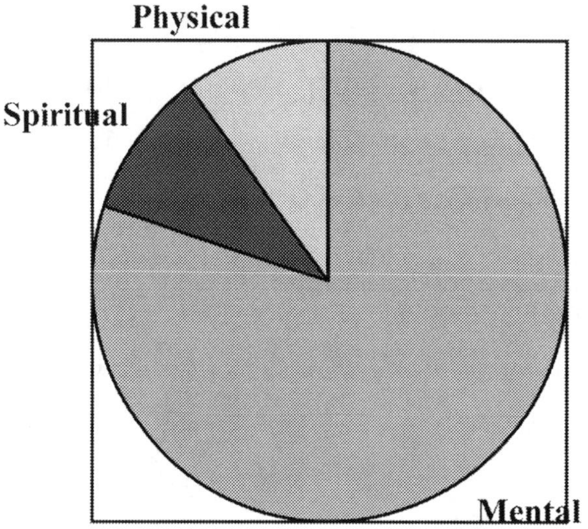

Physical

Spiritual

Mental

Tom is a high school student. His health pie graph below reveals a lot about his health choices and lifestyle.

Utilizing what you have learned in Contract for a Healthy Life and the balancing of health, what conclusions can you make about Tom's health and life by evaluating his pie...

> How does Tom do in school?
>
> How does he do in athletics?
>
> In what hobbies or clubs does he participate?
>
> How does he interact with others?
>
> What kind of friends and friendships does he have?
>
> What are his priorities, strengths, and weaknesses?

> Any other conclusions?

You may have mentioned?

Physical	Mental	Spiritual
Not very active	Very smart	Keeps to himself
Poor diet	Dean's list	Does little for others
Poor sleeping habits	College bound	Has few friends
Eating disorder	Loves solving puzzles	Doesn't express his emotions freely

<u>Step Two:</u> If Tom were to make <u>no</u> changes in his pie, what might his life and health be like in 20 years?

What would he look like?

Where does he live?

What type of job does he have?

What types and kinds of relationships does he have?

What kind of recreation does he participate in?

What are his priorities, strengths, and weaknesses?

Has he developed any diseases or illnesses?

Any other conclusions?

<u>Step Three:</u> We've turned back the hands of time ... and you are now Tom's high school guidance counselor.

You have made an assessment of Tom's current wellness, recognize the need for him to rebalance his health pie graph, and are very knowledgeable about Contract for a Healthy Life and balancing one's health. What advice would you give to him to prevent future health issues and help him on the road to balancing his pie?

Reflect on the conclusions you made earlier and the potential long-term consequences to his life choices. What things might you suggest?

Did you mention...

~ *Involvement in school and community activities*

~ *Support strategies*

~ *Changes in behavior: eating, exercise, and homework habits*

THE POWER OF CHANGE

In reading the lives of great men, I found that the first victory they won was over themselves… self-discipline with all of them came first…

~ Harry S. Truman

THE POWER OF CHANGE

Making the decision to change a behavior might be the most difficult part of change. It is important to know whether it is time to make a change and commit to implementing a contract. Reading this guide with your class is an informative and effective way to begin believing that there is a need for change. Start by having the class ask these questions:

*Why do I need to make a change? Is there a problem?

*What do I want to change?

*What behavior changes will I implement to resolve this problem?

*Am I willing to change?

*How will I benefit from this change?

Next, review a list of pros and cons. Take time to reflect before making these lists. Include the benefits of change and the consequences.

Finally, formulate a vision of the post-change self. Ask students to reflect: Do you look better? Are you in better physical condition, more energetic, happier? Do you feel smarter, more serene, and confident? Often, a vision of the final result will stimulate a reason to change. Once it is decided that an old behavior is not in one's best interest and what change is needed, you're ready for the next step.

Choosing a strategy that is compatible with how you operate is essential for success. Before you select a measurement to record any change, answer the following questions:

- Has it been easy for me to make changes in the past?

- Will my chances for success improve if I make changes gradually, using small steps?

- Do I perform better when there is an abrupt change?

- Where is the best place for me to keep my contract measurement so that I'm sure I will record progress and information daily?

- Should I choose a contract measurement that is simple or do I need to record detailed information?

The Power to Change

Making a decision to change a behavior could be the most difficult part of changing. Knowing whether you want to make a change and if you are ready to commit to change is important before implementing your contract.

First, start by asking yourself these questions:

1. Do I need to change? Is there any area needing improvement?

2. What are some consequences if I don't change?

3. What are some benefits if I do change?

4. What behavior changes will I have to make to resolve this problem?

5. Am I willing to change?

6. What is the major goal I wish to achieve?

CHOOSING A SUPPORT PERSON

The task ahead of us is never as great as the power behind us...

~ Alcoholics Anonymous

MAKING A CONNECTION: CHOOSING A SUPPORT PERSON

Many of us are familiar with the popular TV show *Who Wants to be a Millionaire?* During the show, contestants are allowed to "call a friend" if they don't know the answer to a question. They can choose one person from a pre-selected group, each of whom is knowledgeable in one area of academia. The contestant selects the person he or she feels will provide the correct answer for that particular question. Most often, they choose wisely, the answer is correct, and the contestant moves on to a new level that brings them closer to winning the one million dollars. In this instance the support system set up before the show provides a greater chance for success and often results in a win-win situation. The format used on this show is a great example of a support system that we can follow in our daily lives. Few people know the answers to all questions and problems.

Everyone needs support at different times in life. Without the encouragement of and accountability to a support group or individual, few people are able to sustain long-term lifestyle changes. Turning to another person for help is considered a high-quality behavior that exemplifies spiritual and mental exercise. Knowing where to turn is very important. There are people in our lives from which to choose. People close to us offer a great number of helpful qualities, and when you combine their roles and supportive styles they form part of a three-layer support system called the "Support Team." This "support team" is very useful when we need answers, direction, guidance, and comfort. For example, a family relative may have a strong intellectual background that is useful when asking academic questions. Another may demonstrate great vision or insight in areas of philosophy. Both of these support people offer different types of information and each support style is a valuable resource. There are also people in our lives who share and celebrate our accomplishments. They are there through the most difficult life experiences as well. These are people who are most important. Identifying people and the roles they provide as a support person can help us turn to the right person at the right time. There are three layers of an effective support system. They include the "Primary Support Team," the "Assistance Team," and the "Community Team." Taking time to identify and place individuals in each of these teams provides tremendous resources for our needs and can help to move us in the right direction.

During class discussion we share ideas about the importance of relying on others when we are in need. We also talk about qualities we think are important for us to have when helping others and compare these to people in our lives who are there when we need them. Some of these qualities include patience, understanding, trust, honesty, active listening, experience, maturity, caring, etc. When you turn to someone for help, advice, suggestions, or a good ear, it's important to know what it is you need from them. Make a list of the qualities that are important when you turn to another person for help.

Each person needs to have support people in his or her life who serve as a resource for guidance, information, comfort, and perspective. Choosing the correct support person for the right situation is essential. For example, it may feel comfortable to talk to a sister or brother about family problems but not for advice with a financial matter. Each person can offer a different support style. Recognizing those strengths and seeking the right individual can make the difference between feeling successful or remaining helpless. Choosing a personal "support team" that provides individuals who are effective in all components of health promotes making better decisions, improves interpersonal relationships, and reduces stress. There are 6 roles that are represented in the Primary Support Team or personal "support team." Each of these roles provides the needed qualities and support for various life experiences. These roles include The Nurturer, Comic, Rapper, Professor, Cheerleader, and Confidant. Using these supportive roles helps unravel questions and sort out solutions for a variety of problems.

The Nurturer offers philosophical perspective for issues related to relationships, values, and emotions. Their purpose is to provide insight, clarity, and vision that relate to the problem. They are there to support through hardships and difficult transitions. They can offer positive enlightenment in almost any situation.

The Comic also plays an important role. Humor is such an important ingredient of health because it helps us to feel good. Finding someone who shares your sense of humor provides a type of spiritual rest that is often up- lifting and stress-reducing. It has been said that laughter is the best medicine and research has indicated that there is a lot of truth to this. The Comic can help give an added dimension of relief in difficult situations. The Comic helps to escort us through life with less spiritual waste.

The <u>Professor</u> is a wealth of information. The Professor is someone to seek when the question is intellectual. The Professor enjoys conversing and often knows where to find a solution when he or she doesn't have the answer. The Professor is usually well read, has acquired a proficient vocabulary, and is efficient in a variety of academics.

The <u>Rapper</u> is a person who is easy to talk to. The Rapper can make conversation in most situations, comfortable. The Rapper is a good listener, very approachable, and not intimidating or judgmental toward others.

The <u>Cheerleader </u>wants you to succeed. They cheer for your success and remain enthusiastic when you fail. They are proud of your accomplishments and appreciate your efforts when expectations aren't met. It's clear that the Cheerleader has your best interest at heart and wants to invest in your success. Sharing personal and intimate experiences is comfortable. This person accepts you with your faults and strengths. His or her honesty and guidance encourages you to be the best you can be.

The <u>Confidant</u> plays a wonderful role in our lives. He or she provides unconditional love and often are a parent or sibling. They may fill more than one role in the "Primary Support team." For example a mother can play the role of Cheerleader as well as the Confidant. The Confidant encourages sharing. They are reassuring good listeners. One feels safe when confiding in the Confidant.

It's necessary to fill each of these roles and periodically re-evaluate the "support team," making sure it is still balanced. The "Primary Support Team" consists of individuals we see daily or weekly. They are on call most anytime. The "Primary Support Team" is part of a greater support system that incorporates individuals or groups that we have contact with regularly. An "Assistance Team" is necessary for added support, especially when acceptance with difficult situations is most needed. Often this Assistance Team includes aunts, uncles, grandparents, in-laws, stepsiblings, friends, youth groups, teammates, and neighbors. Their response to a problem can make the difference for an individual who needs to know that they have support and acceptance even when things are not going well.

The third layer of the support system is called the "Community Team." This team is comprised of individuals from the community who offer expertise, education, or suggestions in specific areas of our health. Doctors, psychologists, coaches, teachers, religious leaders and professional support organizations are a few of the supportive roles that provide a resource for information in their field. Society has taught us that it is beneficial to ask professionals, whether it is an individual or group, for help; however, people don't practice this enough.

As your students develop their contracts, ask them to evaluate what type of support they'll need to accomplish their goal. Refer to the visual support team graph and select the person or people who will best help to implement Contract for a Healthy Life. Once the students choose a Primary Support person for their contract, they each schedule time to present their goals and explain what is expected from a support person. First and foremost, they should ask the person if they are willing to be their support person. They should explain that their role is not to make the student reach their goal but to encourage, remind, compliment, and ask how things are going with regard to the contract. They might notice some changes and encourage further progress. They also will sign the student's measuring tool weekly. These measurements are brought in each Friday for added support from the teacher and other classmates.

THE SUPPORT TEAM

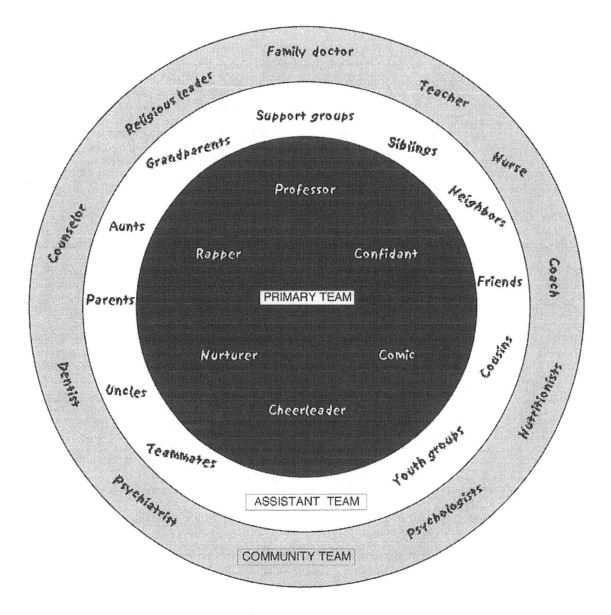

MY SUPPORT TEAM

MY PRIMARY TEAM: People in your daily life with special attributes who offer. you love, comfort, advice, or help.

Cheerleader -   *Professor –*

Confidant -   *Nurturer –*

Rapper -   *Comic –*

ASSISTANCE TEAM: People who you have contact with on a regular basis and play a role in your life.

COMMUNITY TEAM: Professional and community resources who have expertise and can offer education or assistance in a specified field or area.

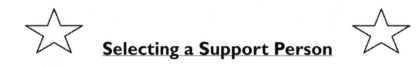

Selecting a Support Person

STEP ONE: Think. Decide which person would be the most effective support person for you.

STEP TWO: Ask this person if they would agree to the following:

1. to <u>listen</u> to your project idea
2. to agree to <u>encourage</u> you, notice any changes, and support your project goals
3. to give advice <u>when asked</u>
4. not to <u>make</u> you do this… it's your project
5. to review and sign measuring tool (log/journal) once a week

STEP THREE: If this person agrees to the conditions above, put his/her name on your contract as your support person.

STUDENT SAMPLES AND INTERVIEW

I LIKE MYSELF NOW

Once you see a child's self-image begin to improve, you will see significant gains in achievement areas, but even more important, you will see a child who is beginning to enjoy life more...
~ Wayne Dyer

Student Samples

I have been teaching the strategies for Contract for a Healthy Life for many years. There are many students who have engaged in this project with great success. I will now share some of these examples. In the preface I shared Jake's story. He is a true example of the success story. As a teacher, it's always rewarding to recognize when students understand and implement their knowledge.

Warren:

As an eighth grade student, Warren's academic performance had deteriorated to the point that he decided his academic failures were too monumental to overcome. At the time he was failing or near-failing all of his academic subjects. He came to second quarter health class with a quiet demeanor and a message that he was in class physically but not mentally or spiritually. As our class discussed the definition of health, I encouraged Warren to participate, but he showed little motivation. When it came time to choose a behavior change, we sat down and talked about some of his interests. I discovered Warren had at one time been a very good math student, but because of personal reasons, all of his grades, including math, were failing. After further discussion Warren agreed to try to improve his math grade by monitoring his mental exercise. Each night he would study math for 15 minutes whether or not he had a test or quiz the next day. He asked his sister, who was very good in math, to be his support person. As a support person, her role is to help when asked and to observe and comment on changes in Warren's math performance. Each week our class briefly shares changes that have been made. Warren rarely offered information during these reviews. One day at an afternoon faculty meeting I overheard a group of eighth grade teachers comparing academic information about a student. Several teachers were very frustrated that this student was still not achieving in their classes and wondered how he had improved so quickly in math. I asked if they were talking about Warren and they said they were. They couldn't figure out why his grade went from an F to a B in math and he was still not performing in other classes. I shared with them that he was using his math class as part of his health project and that this might be one reason for the improvement. I saw Warren the next day and asked him if his math grade was improving. He said it was and he was only studying math a short period of time each night

52

with his sister. I asked him if he felt that his grade improved because he made it part of his health contract and he said it did. For this period of time Warren understood the impact of self-empowerment as he improved his grade and raised his self-esteem. In his final presentation to the class he displayed his signed math papers and grades on his poster. He was pleased with his accomplishment. When we were finished with our quarter, I encouraged Warren to continue planning strategies to improve his other grades and as I followed his progress discovered he did improve by the end of the year.

Garret:

Garret was part of the Guided Learning Program at our middle school. This program is for students who have behavioral difficulties. The purpose of the program is to mainstream students into the regular classroom while supporting both academic and behavioral goals. Eighth grade was the second time I had Garret in health class. We got along great in seventh grade. When Garret first chose his contract strategy, he wanted to change his diet because he ate a lot of junk food and was overweight. Initially he tried this behavior change but quickly became disinterested because he really couldn't notice any immediate changes. We talked about what he could do to notice a change more quickly. Garret and I began to explore frustrations he experienced with his interpersonal relationships. He had a hard time getting along with others and decided to use a point sheet as a measuring tool for his daily behavior. Each teacher signed and evaluated his daily behavior using a number system. For each class he would receive a number from one to four, four being the highest rating for great behavior. Initially Garret was often sent to the dean's office for inappropriate behavior. His point sheet usually had low numbers in each of his classes. We talked about some of the rewards he could experience if he chose to change some of his behaviors. We also discussed how getting along with others might make him feel better both in and out of school. After lengthy discussions, I was pleased when he said he had an idea that might help. He initiated and signed up for 4 anger management sessions with our school psychologist. These sessions offered strategies that Garret might use in school. After 2 weeks I began to notice that the numbers on his point sheet were rising to periodic 3's. He looked better and when he shared his progress with me he sounded more confident. Eventually Garret's point sheet demonstrated that he was interacting much better in his classes and he would receive 3 and 4 points. When he gave his verbal presentation to the class, he said he felt much better about himself and that he was proud of his accomplishment. He used his point sheets to illustrate the progress of his success. Garret shared how his relationships at home had greatly improved and his efforts created a better environment.

Matt:

Matt was a wonderful middle school student with a great heart. Matt had a learning disability and at times this affected his self-esteem. Sometimes Matt would walk down the hallway looking downcast. During his middle school years, Matt received a great deal of support from both classroom and special education teachers. This support made quite a difference over the years and by the time Matt was in eighth grade, he seemed more comfortable. In our health class, Matt decided he wanted to work on his physical exercise to get into better shape and to help lose some extra pounds. He designed a measuring tool that recorded weekly exercises and discoveries. When it came time to share his presentation, Matt seemed a little disappointed that he hadn't reached his goal. When asked what his goal was, he said he wanted to lose 10 pounds but had lost only six. Standing in front of the class, there was a noticeable difference in Matt's physique. He looked thinner and when the class praised him for his commitment to lose the weight, he held his head high and with great confidence. He said he felt great and that even a few pounds made a big difference. He felt confident that he would continue with his plan to reach his goal.

Interview

Dennis:

The following is an interview with one student whose progress and presentation left a lasting impression. Dennis is an eighth grade boy who wanted to make some changes that would improve his physical and spiritual health. During his Contract for a Healthy Life project, his goal was to lose 10 pounds. Here are questions and answers that reflect his progress and ultimate success.

1. What initiated your idea to lose weight during your project?

    A. We were going to be tested for the mile run in a few weeks and I remember that in sixth grade my time was 11 minutes for the mile. I wanted to do much better this year. I wanted to feel comfortable as I ran the final test. I also wanted to be comfortable with myself visually. I felt I needed to lose some weight. I thought this project could improve both my physical health and self-esteem.

2. How did you measure your progress?

    A. I set up a daily exercise program that included push-ups, sit-ups, and lifting weights. I planned to do these each day for the 8 week contract period. At first I did this for only 10 minutes a day. As I gradually improved my fitness, I increased the time to 30 minutes. I used a chart to record the type of exercise, number of repetitions, and intensity of the workout.

3. Who was your support person? How did this work out?

    A. My mom was my support person. She helped me monitor my eating habits. Her support was helpful during the process.

4. When did you first notice a change?

    A. After two weeks I noticed I felt better. I was more comfortable around people. I also noticed that I was moving better in my physical activities in gym and after-school baseball. The main thing was that I felt better, and I liked feeling like that. The first people who noticed and said something to me were family members who thought I looked different and it felt great to hear that. I also remember that toward the end of the project there was a full week when I felt so energized. It was a new feeling and I really liked it. My running on the baseball team improved too. As the contract continued, I kept noticing improvements in both my physical and spiritual health.

5. Do you feel you were successful?

   A. Yes. During the contract time period I lost 6 pounds. Since that time four months ago, I have maintained or lost a little more. My mile run time improved. I ran the final test in 8 minutes and 10 seconds and I felt much more comfortable as I ran it. I feel that my self-esteem has also improved a great deal. I feel better about myself and now know that this project helped me understand that I can accomplish improvements in myself. If I need to change something about myself, I have the ability to do it.

6. What did you learn from this project?

   A. I learned how important it is to stay in shape and to eat healthy. I learned that it is possible to change a weight problem into a lifestyle that keeps you feeling good about yourself. I still watch what I eat and stay away from junk food and sugar. I still exercise. Most importantly, I still feel great about the way I look, feel, and perform. I learned that this process can be used in other health areas and that you have the ability to improve how you feel about yourself.

Exploring Needs with Special Students At Blackham Middle School

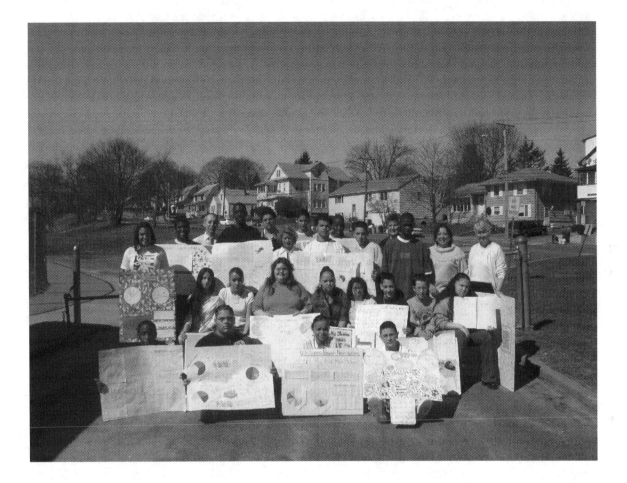

Back Row

Lays, Wayne, Mr. O'Keefe, James, Mrs. Paulette Miller, Paul, Michael, Robert, Darnel, Anthony, Sharon Kowalchik, Evan, Ms.Lorenz, Patty Eng

Middle Row- Seated

Yvette, Denise, Mistylyn, Nicole, Megan, David, Jonathan, Keisha

Floor

Le-Quan, Evander, Kia, Hanser

PROGRAM SUMMARY

I had the privilege of working with students at Read and Blackham Middle Schools in Bridgeport, Connecticut. These are the largest elementary and middle schools in Connecticut, with over 1,500 students. There are no formal health classes in either school. I met social workers Sharon Kowalchik and Patty Eng, who work at Read and Blackham Middle Schools in Bridgeport. They counsel at-risk students. They counsel many students with a variety of health issues, and we felt this was a perfect place to implement Contract for a Healthy Life. Sharon and Patty are dedicated educators, and their willingness to explore and pursue this in a classroom setting was instrumental in the program's development.

The class selected for this program is a seventh and eighth grade self-contained inclusion classroom. In this class there are 21 students who have a variety of special needs that are addressed daily. Classroom teachers Paulette Miller and Gary O'Keefe assisted Patty Eng as she introduced the language and concept of Contract for a Healthy Life. As students became familiar with the idea of improving their lives, each chose to improve one part of their physical, mental, or spiritual health. They filled out the paperwork, selected a support person and measuring tool, and began their journey for the next three months. Because this is a contained classroom, students were able to extend their time frame and continued their goals for 3-4 months. Patty Eng facilitated their progress during weekly sessions in their classroom.

I returned to listen to the students' presentations and was extremely impressed with their final summaries. I found their choice of goals especially interesting because some were unique to their environment. As I entered the room I sensed pride and accomplishment among the students. They were very eager to share their stories and projects. Here are some examples of these presentations.

Denise, Anthony, Nicole, James, and Keisha all used measuring tools and support people to help them turn back their clock and get more rest. Each felt the lack of sleep was interfering with their grades, relationships, and self-esteem. As each increased the number of hours of sleep each night, they discovered that they changed more than just their physical health. Their spiritual and mental health had improved as well. There were also a number of students whose goals were to lose weight or to get into better physical shape. Each chose a routine and support person that enabled him or her to make progress toward the goal. Another student found it difficult to get to school regularly. Truancy was becoming a serious problem. With adult support and guidance, this student chose coming to school as a goal for her contract. Her attendance improved markedly and she is now working on goals in other areas of her health.

STUDENT SAMPLES

1. Robert chose to make a change to his physical health because he felt he was too big for his age, and this made him feel uncomfortable in school. Robert weighed 235 pounds as an eighth grade student. He listened to Mrs. Patty share the information and project goals and decided he wanted to try to change his appearance. Robert began an exercise program. He walked at the high school track 5 days a week for 35 minutes each day and watched his diet. He filled in his daily chart every night and checked in with his cousin Sammy, who was his support person. His teachers were also helpful in supporting Robert as he reached his goal. Robert lost over 37 pounds. When asked what he learned about himself, he said he learned that he has the power to motivate himself to do something that will make him feel better. He knows how to commit to a wonderful habit and make it part of his life. Robert is now a support person for a teacher's aid who is trying to lose weight.

2. Paul wanted to make a change to the spiritual part of his health. Paul felt that his complaining contributed to the poor relationship he had with his stepfather. Paul decided he would stop complaining at home when asked to do a chore. He even started to do chores before he was asked. Paul used a calendar to record his findings. He asked his stepfather to be his support person. Paul worked on this for two months and found that his project helped him become a more approachable person. People liked him better and treated him better. Paul says that now he gets along so well with his stepfather that they do a lot of fun things together. Paul was able to change his spiritual health while improving his relationship with his stepfather.

3. Le-Quan was having difficulty managing pain he felt from a bladder condition that caused kidney stones. It is difficult for him to go through a day without this pain. Le-Quan decided to try to change his physical health by changing some of his habits. Drinking water is most important when afflicted with this condition. For his project he decided to stop drinking soda and start drinking more water. He marked the calendar every time he drank a glass of water. Over time Le-Quan noticed his pain

was becoming more manageable. He will continue with this project and hopes further treatments will help heal his health condition.

4. Meghan decided to make a change to her spiritual health. Meghan has felt anger and sadness with her limited physical mobility and compromised respiration since birth. Meghan wrote her feelings in a journal every day and recorded her entries on a chart. As I read through her journal, I sensed that while using this method to explore her frustrations, Meg felt both empowered and comforted. She learned that writing in her journal every day helps manage frustration and anger, especially when others hurt her feelings. Meghan said her grandmother was a very good support person and she'll continue this project because it has made her feel much better.

5. Jonathon was not doing his homework, and he admitted that he would have better grades if he did his homework every night. Jonathon used a homework chart to record his completed homework assignments and discovered that he felt better about school as he improved his grades. He learned that if you get in the habit of doing your homework, you could improve your mental health. Feeling better in school improved Jonathon's spiritual health too. He discovered that others treat him with more respect when he does better in school.

6. Yvette also wanted to improve her grades and began studying more before tests and quizzes. She used a calendar to record test dates. This helped her remember when the tests were scheduled and projects were due. Yvette asked her mom to be her support person. Yvette discovered that studying really works. Yvette's teacher agrees. Yvette's grades have improved and she has become a better student. Yvette also found that she felt better about herself because she was able to stick to her commitment and improve her grades.

As the presentations finished I felt extremely happy for each of these students. All were able to succeed in all or part of his or her goals. They shared experiences with a sense of empowerment and felt they had made a difference that would encourage them to make choices toward a healthier lifestyle. Most impressive was their ability to define empowerment and the strong impact it can have toward improving their health.

Contract for a Healthy Life will continue at Blackham Middle School. Plans to establish this program at the elementary level using older students as support persons is now being proposed. I will continue my new friendship with Bridgeport schools while learning how this program can grow and improve other populations. I found this experience to be one of the most rewarding teaching experiences of my career.

SUMMARY

The sense of duty to continue is present in all of us. A duty to strive is the duty of us all. I felt a call to that duty...

~ Abraham Lincoln

SUMMARY

Contract for a Healthy Life began as part of a class discussion while trying to develop a common definition of health. Since that class 19 years ago, this program has developed into one that has helped improve the health of many adolescents. Prior to this assignment, these students believed that their primary resource for healing or rebalancing their health was with outside sources such as their physician, parents, counselors, etc. If they did not feel well, it was up to someone else to fix them. These resources are valuable in many ways and we do encourage students to seek help from adults rather than resorting to low-quality fixes such as drugs or other high- risk behaviors. It is important for them to realize that to do nothing when their health is in need of improvement can be very detrimental to their health. It is most important to teach our young children that they also can make a difference in their own health. Recognizing and adjusting behaviors that interfere with our health can prevent future illnesses, failures, and even shortened life expectancy. With guidance, these students have taken a journey in which they reflect on their own physical, mental, and spiritual health and take action to improve behaviors that can help them to feel better physically, mentally, and spiritually. Increasing sleep, managing anger and stress, and improving grades in school are some of the ways these students have helped themselves. Defining health, using the wellness survey to assess their own health, identifying the need for change, and choosing a support person and measuring tool to record changes are the strategies that have helped these students to succeed. Understanding and implementing the power they have to make and sustain these changes is life altering.

Health and science teachers have implemented this program in eighth grade middle schools. Social workers in urban schools have also used this program for at-risk students whose needs are not being met at home. Contract for a Healthy Life is a program that can be modified for elementary and high school students as well as individual adults, recovering addicts, and hospital patients. These strategies are also used as a guide for family reflection and to identify goals that can improve home life.

A perfectly balanced health pie graph is difficult to sustain because the nature and flow of life contributes consistent fluctuations and challenges in physical, mental and spiritual health. Many students now understand that with education, support, and vision, anyone can maintain optimal health.

TEACHER MATERIALS

- Lesson Development

- Contract Brochure

- Wellness Survey Pre-Test and Post-Test Worksheets

- Modified Wellness Survey

- Goal-setting Guidelines

- Contract Form

- Support Person Agreement and Evaluation

- Sample Measuring Tools

- Visual and Oral Presentation Guidelines

Lesson Development

1. Introduction and definition of Health ~ Define Physical, Mental and Spiritual Health using a pie graph. Identify 4 daily requirements, Food, Rest, Exercise and Elimination and apply to each health component. Include high and low-quality behaviors. Distribute Contract Brochure. (Can be signed by parent) *Worksheet Provided

2. Visual Activity ~ Share and examine Tom and Sally's health journey from high school through adulthood. Add an activity for students to explore suggestions that may help Tom and Sally's future. Identify student's personal pie graph to illustrate individual physical, mental and spiritual health. Identify health behaviors that reflect pie graph.

3. Wellness Survey ~ Pre-test; students assess their own health using the wellness survey. Apply results to bar and/or pie graph. Discuss strengths and weaknesses.

4. Examine Goal-Setting graph ~ Identify strategies to manage, improve, increase and reduce health behaviors. Identify personal physical, mental, and spiritual goals for improvement. Research data related to selected area of health for personal improvement. * Worksheet Provided

5. Complete and sign Contract form. ~ Identify value of support person and qualities needed for success. Identify support person for Contract project.

6. Introduce measuring tools. ~ Select measuring tool to be signed weekly by support person.

7. Wellness survey ~ Post-test; students re-take the wellness survey and compare results with pre-test graph information.

8. Identify required criteria for final verbal and visual class presentation. ~ Review reflection questions. Share poster examples. Review evaluation forms signed by support person.

9. Review teacher evaluation. ~ Examine Contract rubric with class.

10. Student Presentations

RESEARCH DATA INFORMATION WORKSHEET

ARTICLE SUMMARY & REVIEW

Research information that will provide useful facts related to your personal contract and goal

Student Name: _____ Per. _____

Area of Health Working on: _____

Contract Goal: _____

TITLE OF ARTICLE: _____

SOURCE (WEBSITE OR MAGAZINE): _____

1. Briefly summarize the key points in the article:

2. What did you learn that may help you with your contract goal (any information or skills)?

CONTRACT BROCHURE

Copy the following two pages back to back to create a 3-fold student brochure

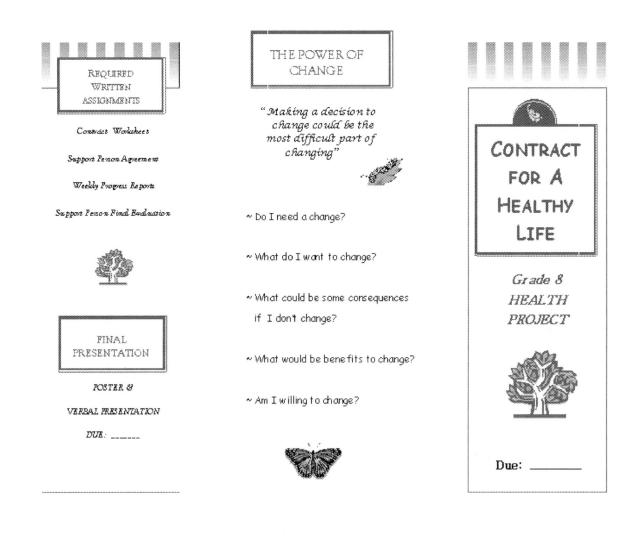

REQUIRED WRITTEN ASSIGNMENTS

Contract Worksheet

Support Person Agreement

Weekly Progress Reports

Support Person Final Evaluation

FINAL PRESENTATION

POSTER &

VERBAL PRESENTATION

DUE: _____

THE POWER OF CHANGE

"Making a decision to change could be the most difficult part of changing"

~ Do I need a change?

~ What do I want to change?

~ What could be some consequences if I don't change?

~ What would be benefits to change?

~ Am I willing to change?

CONTRACT FOR A HEALTHY LIFE

Grade 8 HEALTH PROJECT

Due: _____

PROJECT DESCRIPTION

You will create a health goal and design a 6-8 week plan to measure and assess your progress.

PROCEDURES

1. Create a current health profile.
2. Develop a goal and strategies to improve your physical, mental, or spiritual health.
3. Design a measuring tool to record your progress.
4. Select a support person and establish guidelines. Report your progress and setbacks to this person.
5. Create a visual presentation: a poster.
6. Deliver an oral presentation to class.

BALANCING YOUR HEALTH

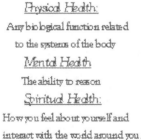

Physical Health:
Any biological function related to the systems of the body
Mental Health
The ability to reason
Spiritual Health:
How you feel about yourself and interact with the world around you.

Your success can be enhanced by good use of your support person...

A SUPPORT PERSON...

~ *Listens*

~ *Notices changes*

~ *Offers suggestions*

~ *Allows student to be in control*

~ *Reviews and signs Weekly Progress Reports*

Contract for a Healthy Life

SURVEY PACKET

Survey Questions
Evaluation Graphs and Worksheets

Student Name:_____

Period:__

My Wellness Survey

In this survey you will be exploring your personal health as you answer questions about your health-related behaviors and decisions. There will be questions on all the "12 ingredients of health".

The questions are designed to categorize and assess the quality of your behaviors and decisions as they relate to health. This is a tool that can identify your strong and weak areas of health.

You will use the survey results to complete a health summary page and then create a graph that illustrates a visual and comprehensive profile of your current wellness. When your contract is ready for presentation, take the wellness survey again as a post-test and compare the results to your pre-test summaries. Review results and then begin preparing for your final verbal and visual class presentations.

DIRECTIONS:

STEP ONE: Answer the questions on all the survey pages and record your results on the first line next to each question. You must rank each answer to every question from 0 to 4. Please try to be as accurate and honest as possible.

STEP TWO: When you finish the questionnaire, tally numbers on each page and plot the results on both the bar and pie graph.

STEP THREE: Answer the questions on the Survey Results worksheet.

STEP FOUR: When you are ready to complete your contract and present to the class, re-take the wellness survey and record results on the second line provided next to each question.

PHYSICAL FOOD

After each question, write the number that corresponds with the answer that is most true.

NEVER = 0 points

SELDOM to RARELY = 1 point

SOMETIMES = 2 points

OFTEN to FREQUENTLY = 3 points

ALWAYS = 4 points

<u>PRE</u>   <u>POST</u>

1. DO YOU EAT A HEALTHY BREAKFAST?   _____   _____

2. DO YOU LIMIT INTAKE OF PRODUCTS WITH SUGAR?   _____   _____

3. DO YOU TAKE DAILY SUPPLEMENTS?   _____   _____
   (VITAMINS, MINERALS, ETC?)

4. DO YOU MAKE EATING DECISIONS BASED ON READING N UTRITION LABELS ON PACKAGED FOOD?   _____   _____

5. DO YOU EAT AT LEAST 2 SERVINGS OF BOTH FRUITS AND VEGETABLES DAILY?   _____   _____

6. DO YOU TRACK YOUR DAILY INTAKE OF CALORIES, PROTEINS AND CARBOHYDRATES?   _____   _____

7. DO YOU DRINK AT LEAST 6 GLASSES OF WATER DAILY?   _____   _____

8. DO YOU HAVE 2 SERVINGS OF CALCIUM DAILY?   _____   _____

9. DO YOU EAT AT LEAST 3 MEALS EACH DAY?   _____   _____

10. DO YOU LIMIT YOUR INTAKE OF FATTY FOODS?   _____   _____

PHYSICAL REST

> After each question, write the number that corresponds with the answer that is most true.
>
> NEVER = 0 points
>
> SELDOM to RARELY = 1 point
>
> SOMETIMES = 2 points
>
> OFTEN to FREQUENTLY = 3 points
>
> ALWAYS = 4 points

PRE POST

1. DO YOU GET 9 to 9 ½ HOURS OF SLEEP PER NIGHT? _____ _____

2. DO YOU FALL ASLEEP EASILY? _____ _____

3. IS YOUR SLEEP CONTINUOUS (UNINTERRUPTED)? _____ _____

4. DO YOU WAKE UP EASILY AND FEEL RESTED? _____ _____

5. DO YOU PERFORM BETTER ON TESTS AND WRITTEN ASSESSMENTS AFTER A GOOD NIGHT'S SLEEP? _____ _____

6. DOES YOUR AMOUNT OF REST AFFECT YOUR INTERPERSONAL RELATIONSHIPS? _____ _____

7. DO YOU PERFORM BETTER IN PHYSICAL ACTIVITIES AFTER A GOOD NIGHT'S SLEEP? _____ _____

8. DO YOU FEEL WELL RESTED AND ENERGIZED AFTER 8-9 HOURS OF SLEEP?? _____ _____

9. DO YOU PURPOSEFULLY REST WHEN YOU ARE TIRED? _____ _____

10. WHEN YOU HAVE HAD A GOOD NIGHT'S SLEEP, DO YOU PARTICIPATE MORE IN YOUR CLASSES? _____ _____

PHYSICAL EXERCISE

After each question, write the number that corresponds with the answer that is most true.

NEVER = 0 points

SELDOM to RARELY = 1 point

SOMETIMES = 2 points

OFTEN to FREQUENTLY = 3 points

ALWAYS = 4 points

1. DO YOU EXERCISE VIGOROUSLY AT LEAST 30 MINUTES, 3 TO 5 DAYS A WEEK? _____ _____

2. DO YOU WARM UP BEFORE A PHYSICAL ACTIVITY? _____ _____

3. DO YOU USUALLY COOL-DOWN AFTER A PHYSICAL ACTIVITY? _____ _____

4. DO YOU PARTICIPATE IN A ROUTINE FLEXIBILITY AND/OR STRENGTH PROGRAM? _____ _____

5. DO YOU PARTICIPATE IN ANY AFTER SCHOOL PHYSICAL ACTIVITY OR SPORT? _____ _____

6. CAN YOU RUN THE MILE IN 10 MINUTES OR LESS? _____ _____

7. DO YOU WEAR PROPER CLOTHING AND FOOTWEAR WHILE EXERCISING? _____ _____

8. DO YOU WEAR SUN PROTECTION WHEN OUTSIDE FOR AN EXTENDED PERIOD OF TIME? _____ _____

9. DO YOU WEAR PROTECTIVE GEAR (HELMET, SEATBELT, ETC)? _____ _____

10. DO YOU KNOW YOUR RESTING HEART RATE? _____ _____

PHYSICAL ELIMINATION

After each question, write the number that corresponds with the answer that is most true.

NEVER = 0 points

SELDOM to RARELY = 1 point

SOMETIMES = 2 points

OFTEN to FREQUENTLY = 3 points

ALWAYS = 4 points

1. DO YOU SHOWER AT LEAST EVERY OTHER DAY? _____ _____

2. DO YOU SUFFER FROM A COLD 2 TIMES OR FEWER PER YEAR? _____ _____

3. ARE YOU WITHIN THE NORMAL WEIGHT RANGE FOR YOUR AGE? _____ _____

4. DO YOU WASH YOUR HANDS AT LEAST 5-6 TIMES A DAY? _____ _____

5. DO YOU BRUSH YOUR TEETH AT LEAST TWICE A DAY? _____ _____

6. DO YOU FLOSS YOUR TEETH DAILY? _____ _____

7. DO YOU USE MOUTHWASH DAILY? _____ _____

8. DO YOU USE A NAIL CLIPPER TO MAINTAIN YOUR NAILS? _____ _____

9. DO YOU SWEAT A NORMAL AMOUNT WHEN HOT FROM WORKING OUT OR EXERCISING? _____ _____

10. DO YOU HAVE NORMAL FREQUENCY OF URINATION AND BOWEL MOVEMENTS? _____ _____

PHYSICAL HEALTH SUMMARY PAGE

Daily Requirement   Pre-Score   Post-Score

PHYSICAL FOOD =   _____   _____

PHYSICAL REST =   _____   _____

PHYSICAL EXERCISE =   _____   _____

PHYSICAL ELIMINATION =   _____   _____

PHYSICAL HEALTH SUBTOTAL =

PRE-SCORE	POST- SCORE

MENTAL FOOD

After each question, write the number that corresponds with the answer that is most true.

NEVER = 0 points

SELDOM to RARELY = 1 point

SOMETIMES = 2 points

OFTEN to FREQUENTLY = 3 points

ALWAYS = 4 points

1. DO YOU ENJOY READING? _____ _____

2. DO YOU READ FOR ENJOYMENT AT LEAST 3 TIMES
    PER WEEK? _____ _____

3. DO YOU REFLECT IN A JOURNAL OR DIARY? _____ _____

4. DO YOU REGULARLY COMPLETE YOUR HOMEWORK ASSIGNMENTS ON
    TIME? _____ _____

5. DO YOU ENJOY LEARNING NEW THINGS? _____ _____

6. DO YOU KNOW YOUR STRONGEST LEARNING STYLE (HEARING, SEEING,
    OR DOING)? _____ _____

7. DO YOU CONSIDER YOURSELF A GOOD LISTENER? _____ _____

8. DO YOU LIKE TO ASK QUESTIONS ABOUT THINGS YOU ARE NOT SURE OF?

9. ARE YOU SATISFIED WITH YOUR GRADES? _____ _____

10. DO YOU FEEL YOU HAVE SOLID STUDY HABITS? _____ _____

MENTAL REST

After each question, write the number that corresponds with the answer that is most true.

NEVER = 0 points

SELDOM to RARELY = 1 point

SOMETIMES = 2 points

OFTEN to FREQUENTLY = 3 points

ALWAYS = 4 points

1. DO YOU TAKE A BREAK WHEN YOU ARE OVERWHELMED? _____ _____

2. HAVE YOU EVER TRIED MEDITATION, YOGA, OR A RELAXATION PROGRAM? _____ _____

3. DO YOU HAVE A STRATEGY TO HELP REDUCE YOUR STRESS WHEN YOU FEEL STRESSED OUT? _____ _____

4. DO YOU ENJOY FAMILY OUTINGS AND VACATIONS? _____ _____

5. DO YOU LOOK FORWARD TO "FREE TIME" AND YOUR WEEKENDS? _____ _____

6. DO YOU BALANCE YOUR TIME WITH FRIENDS AND FAMILY AND WORK? _____ _____

7. DO YOU EXERCISE REGULARLY FOR ENJOYMENT OR STRESS REDUCTION? _____ _____

8. DO YOU INCLUDE SOME FORM OF MENTAL RELAXATION DAILY? _____ _____

9. ARE YOU COMFORTABLE ABOUT EXPECTATIONS OTHERS HAVE FOR YOU? _____ _____

10. ARE YOU SATISFIED WITH YOUR ACCOMPLISHMENTS? _____ _____

MENTAL EXERCISE

After each question, write the number that corresponds with the answer that is most true.

NEVER = 0 points

SELDOM to RARELY = 1 point

SOMETIMES = 2 points

OFTEN to FREQUENTLY = 3 points

ALWAYS = 4 points

1. DO YOU STUDY THE MATERIAL MORE THAN ONCE BEFORE A TEST OR QUIZ? _____ _____

2. DO YOU REVIEW YOUR ASSIGNMENTS BEFORE YOU HAND THEM IN? _____ _____

3. HAVE YOU EVER MADE A LIST OF PROS AND CONS WHEN STRUGGLING WITH A PROBLEM? _____ _____

4. DO YOU ACTIVELY PARTICIPATE IN EACH CLASS? _____ _____

5. WHEN YOU MISS A CLASS, DO YOU ASK YOUR TEACHER FOR THE INFORMATION YOU MISSED? _____ _____

6. DO YOU STOP TO CONSIDER POSSIBLE CONSEQUENCES BEFORE MAKING A DECISION? _____ _____

7. ARE YOU ORGANIZED WHEN YOU COME TO SCHOOL? _____ _____

8. DO YOU KEEP A DAILY ASSIGNMENT AGENDA OR LIST? _____ _____

9. DO YOU HAVE A SET ROUTINE AND PLACE FOR DOING YOUR HOMEWORK? _____ _____

10. DO YOU FEEL YOU HAVE SOLID STUDY HABITS? _____ _____

MENTAL ELIMINATION

After each question, write the number that corresponds with the answer that is most true.
NEVER = 0 points
SELDOM to RARELY = 1 point
SOMETIMES = 2 points
OFTEN to FREQUENTLY = 3 points
ALWAYS = 4 points

1. DO YOU CORRECT WRONG ANSWERS AND INCORRECT INFORMATION ON TESTS AND QUIZZES? _____ _____

2. DO YOU EASILY REMEMBER REQUIRED FACTS AND INFORMATION? _____ _____

3. DO YOU SEEK ADVICE FROM AN ADULT REGARDING DIFFICULT DECISIONS? _____ _____

4. DO YOU ASK QUESTIONS IN CLASS WHEN YOU ARE CONFUSED? _____ _____

5. ONCE YOU MAKE A TOUGH DECISION, DO YOU STOP WORRYING ABOUT THE OTHER CHOICES? _____ _____

MENTAL HEALTH SUMMARY PAGE

Daily Requirement   Pre-Score   Post-Score

MENTAL FOOD =   _____   _____

MENTAL REST =   _____   _____

MENTAL EXERCISE =   _____   _____

MENTAL ELIMINATION =   _____   _____

MENTAL HEALTH SUBTOTAL =

PRE-SCORE   POST- SCORE

SPIRITUAL FOOD

After each question, write the number that corresponds with the answer that is most true.

NEVER = 0 points

SELDOM to RARELY = 1 point

SOMETIMES = 2 points

OFTEN to FREQUENTLY = 3 points

ALWAYS = 4 points

1. DO YOU HAVE SEVERAL PEOPLE YOU CAN TURN TO FOR SUPPORT (A SUPPORT TEAM)? _____ _____

2. ARE YOU PART OF SOMEONE ELSE'S SUPPORT TEAM? _____ _____

3. DO YOU HAVE ONE ADULT THAT YOU FEEL COMFORTABLE TALKING TO? _____ _____

4. DO YOU FEEL YOU HAVE HAD IMPORTANT ACCOMPLISHMENTS? _____ _____

5. DO YOU FEEL CONFIDENT THAT YOU MAKE POSITIVE DECISIONS FOR YOURSELF? _____ _____

6. DO YOU FEEL GOOD ABOUT YOURSELF? _____ _____

7. DOES YOUR FAMILY MAKE A DAILY EFFORT TO SPEND QUALITY TIME TOGETHER? _____ _____

8. DO YOU RECOGNIZE OTHERS' ACCOMPLISHMENTS? _____ _____

9. DO YOU TURN TO OTHERS FOR SUPPORT? _____ _____

10. DO YOU FEEL LOVED? _____ _____

SPIRITUAL REST

After each question, write the number that corresponds with the answer that is most true.

NEVER = 0 points

SELDOM to RARELY = 1 point

SOMETIMES = 2 points

OFTEN to FREQUENTLY = 3 points

ALWAYS = 4 points

1. DO YOU ALLOW OTHERS TO HELP YOU WHEN YOU ARE IN NEED? _____ _____

2. DO YOU USE PRAYER OR MEDITATION AS A TOOL FOR COMFORT? _____ _____

3. DO YOU OCCASIONALLY DO SOMETHING SPECIAL FOR YOURSELF? _____ _____

4. DO YOU TALK TO SOMEONE WHEN YOU ARE AFRAID? _____ _____

5. DO YOU ENJOY BEING BY YOURSELF AT TIMES? _____ _____

SPIRITUAL EXERCISE

After each question, write the number that corresponds with the answer that is most true.

NEVER = 0 points

SELDOM to RARELY = 1 point

SOMETIMES = 2 points

OFTEN to FREQUENTLY = 3 points

ALWAYS = 4 points

1. DO YOU ENJOY DOING THINGS FOR OTHERS, WITHOUT EXPECTING ANYTHING IN RETURN? _____ _____

2. DO YOU REGULARLY TAKE RESPONSIBILITY FOR ANOTHER PERSON (YOUNGER SIBLING OR FRIEND) OR A PET? _____ _____

3. DO YOU GET ALONG WITH OTHER FAMILY MEMBERS? _____ _____

4. DO YOU LISTEN WITHOUT INTERRUPTION WHEN OTHERS SPEAK? _____ _____

5. DO YOU EASILY FORGIVE YOURSELF WHEN YOU MAKE A MISTAKE? _____ _____

6. DO YOU TALK TO A GUIDANCE COUNSELOR OR AN ADULT WHEN YOU ARE TROUBLED? _____ _____

7. DO YOU EXPRESS YOUR FEELINGS IN A JOURNAL OR DIARY, IN ART, OR IN SONG LYRICS? _____ _____

8. DO YOU FIND IT EASY TO RESOLVE CONFLICTS AND DISPUTES WITH OTHERS? _____ _____

9. DO YOU VOLUNTEER OR PARTICIPATE IN ANY COMMUNITY SERVICE ACTIVITIES? _____ _____

10. AT HOME DO YOU DO CHORES OR TASKS TO HELP WITHOUT BEING ASKED? _____ _____

SPIRITUAL ELIMINATION

After each question, write the number that corresponds with the answer that is most true.

NEVER = 0 points

SELDOM to RARELY = 1 point

SOMETIMES = 2 points

OFTEN to FREQUENTLY = 3 points

ALWAYS = 4 points

1. DO YOU FIND IT EASY TO FORGIVE OTHERS? _____ _____

2. DO YOU PREFER A CONFLICT RESOLUTION THAT BENEFITS BOTH YOU AND THE OTHER PERSON? _____ _____

3. DO YOU REMAIN CALM AND IN CONTROL DURING ARGUMENTS? _____ _____

4. DO YOU WORK TO UNDERSTAND OTHER PEOPLE'S OPINIONS AND POINTS OF VIEW? _____ _____

5. CAN YOU ACCEPT OTHER PEOPLE'S POINT OF VIEW, IF DIFFERENT, WITHOUT TRYING TO PERSUADE THEM TO YOUR WAY OF THINKING? _____ _____

6. CAN YOU ENJOY OTHER PEOPLE'S SUCCESSES WITHOUT FEELING JEALOUS? _____ _____

7. DO YOU LOOK FOR THE BRIGHT SIDE OF LIFE? _____ _____

8. DO YOU TELL SOMEONE WHEN YOU ARE UPSET WITH (HIM/HER) AND WHY? _____ _____

9. DO YOU FIND IT COMFORTABLE TO SAY THAT YOU ARE SORRY WHEN YOU HAVE DONE SOMETHING WRONG? _____ _____

10. ONCE AN ARGUMENT IS OVER, DO YOU MOVE AHEAD WITHOUT ANY BITTERNESS? _____ _____

SPIRITUAL HEALTH SUMMARY PAGE

Daily Requirement	Pre-Score	Post-Score
SPIRITUAL FOOD =	_____	_____
SPIRITUAL REST =	_____	_____
SPIRITUAL EXERCISE =	_____	_____
SPIRITUAL ELIMINATION =	_____	_____

SPIRITUAL HEALTH SUBTOTAL =

PRE-SCORE	POST- SCORE

MY WELLNESS SURVEY RESULTS

Directions: Use each health component's summary page to complete the chart below.

	BEFORE PROJECT (Pre-test)	AFTER PROJECT (Post-test)
PHYSICAL		
Food		
Rest		
Exercise		
Elimination		
Total=		
MENTAL		
Food		
Rest		
Exercise		
Elimination		
Total=		
SPIRITUAL		
Food		
Rest		
Exercise		
Elimination		
Total=		
OVERALLTOTAL=	(Pre-test)	(Post-test)

WELLNESS SURVEY RESULTS: Bar Graph

Directions:
1. Take the information from each summary page and plot your scores in the columns below.
2. Color the boxes going up vertically. Begin at the baseline and continue up to the point where your score would fall.
3. Lastly, add the total scores from all the summary pages and plot that score in the GRAND TOTAL column to get information about your overall wellness.

PHYSICAL HEALTH

FOOD	REST	EXERCISE	ELIMINATION
40	40	40	40
35	35	35	35
30	30	30	30
25	25	25	25
15	15	15	15
0	0	0	

MENTAL HEALTH

FOOD	REST	EXERCISE	ELIMINATION
40	40	40	20
35	35	35	17
30	30	30	13
25	25	25	10
15	15	15	7
0	0	0	

SPIRITUAL HEALTH

FOOD	REST	EXERCISE	ELIMINATION
40	20	40	40
35	17	35	35
30	13	30	30
25	10	25	25
15	7	15	15
0	0	0	0

*scores under the shaded bar indicate areas where improvement is needed!

SAMPLE

FOOD=30
REST=33
EXERCISE=38
ELIMINATION=27

GRAND TOTAL SCORE

What does this tell me about my overall wellness?

415 — TERRIFIC! This is a high level of wellness.

370 — VERY GOOD! Shows good decision making but continue to work on your weak areas.

330 — GOOD! You can raise your levels if you make a few changes.

245 — NEED IMPROVEMENT! You need more information and better decision making skills.

165 — You need to make major changes in your current lifestyle.

BEFORE

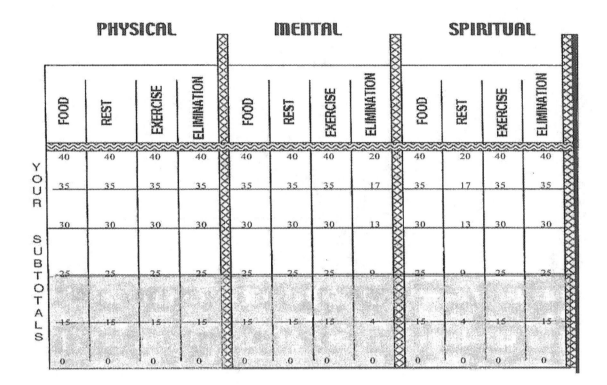

AFTER

Cathleen Hamill

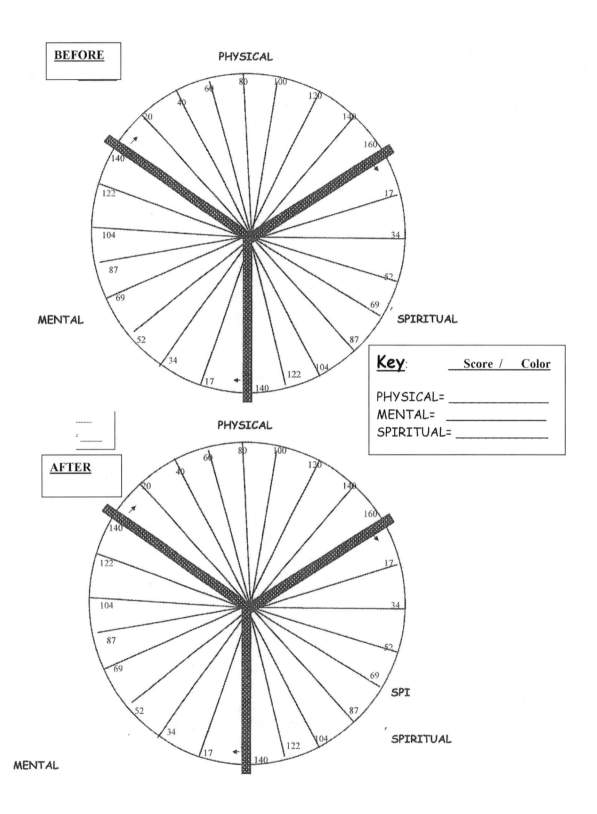

WELLNESS SURVEY RESULTS: Pie Graph

Directions:
1. Take the information from each summary page and plug the total score into the "My Scores" key.
2. Using the scores in the key. Starting at 0, color in the direction of the arrow until you get to where the score would fall.

SAMPLE

PHYSICAL= 140
MENTAL= 100
SPIRITUAL= 100

MENTAL

PHYSICAL

SPIRITUAL

MY SCORES:
PHYSICAL= ____
MENTAL= ____
SPIRITUAL= ____

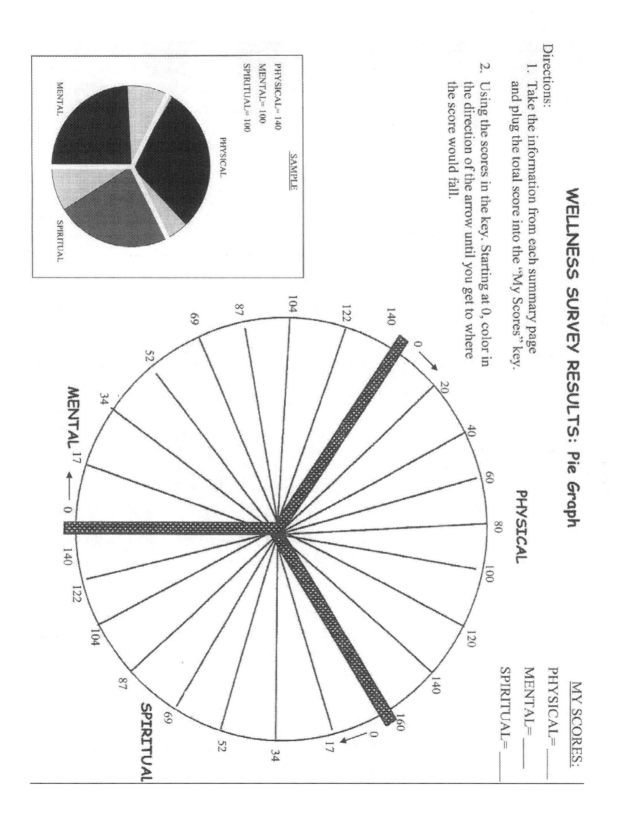

WELLNESS SURVEY WORKSHEET

<u>Directions:</u> Use your survey and graph results to fill in the information requested.

1. My total wellness ranking on the bar graph is: (circle one)

    TERRIFIC   VERY GOOD GOOD   NEEDS IMPROVEMENT   POOR

2. The two areas of health I think are my strongest areas are:
    (Physical, Mental, or Spiritual)

    _____and _____

3. My weakest health area is _____ and the two daily requirements
    that need the most improvement are

    _____and _____

4. Here are three realistic and specific behavior changes I can make to improve my
    wellness level. (e.g., drink more water daily, read 10 minutes more daily, say I'm sorry
    more often)

    _____

    _____

    _____

EVALUATING YOUR SURVEY RESULTS

Your Name: _____ Date:_____

The Interviewer: _____

1. Was your overall wellness rating acceptable to you?
   Yes or No: Explain why or why not.

2. Which overall area of health – physical, mental, or spiritual – scored highest?
   And which daily requirement scored highest?

3. Which overall area of health – physical, mental, or spiritual –scored lowest?
   And which daily requirement scored lowest?

4. Which area of your health do <u>you</u> think needs to be changed and how? (increased, modified, reduced)

5. What are some consequences if you don't change?

6. What are some benefits if you change?

7. What other benefits would you gain if you did change? *(happier, in better physical shape, get along better with others, more energetic, more confident, smarter)*

CONTRACT FOR A HEALTHY LIFE RESEARCH

Student Name: _____

Internet Resource(s)= _____(ATTACH
ARTICLE IF POSSIBLE)

Suggested Sites:

www.educationplanner.org/students/self-assessments   www.studygs.net/
index.htm

www.kidshealth.org www.helpguide.org www.nih.org www.myplate.gov

WHAT DID YOU LEARN?

HOW WILL THIS HELP YOU AND YOUR PROJECT?

MODIFIED WELLNESS SURVEY

PHYSICAL, MENTAL, SPIRITUAL

FOOD, REST, EXERCISE, ELIMINATION

After each question, write the number that corresponds with the answer that is most true.

NEVER = 0 points

SELDOM to RARELY = 1 point

SOMETIMES = 2 points

OFTEN to FREQUENTLY = 3 points

ALWAYS = 4 points

PHYSICAL FOOD

1. Do you eat breakfast everyday? _____ _____

2. Do you eat at least one piece of fruit everyday? _____ _____

3. Do you eat at least 2 servings of vegetables everyday? _____ _____

4. Do you drink at least 8 glasses of water a day? _____ _____

PHYSICAL REST

1. Do you sleep 9 or more hours a day? _____ _____

2. Do you fall asleep easily? _____ _____

3. Do you wake up easily and feel rested? _____ _____

4. Do you stop and relax when you are tired? _____ _____

PHYSICAL EXERCISE

1. Do you exercise more than 3 times a week? _____ _____

2. Do you do warm-up stretches and exercises before exercising? _____

3. Do you do cool-down exercises after exercising? _____ _____

4. Do you run do 5 or more push-ups? _____ _____

PHYSICAL ELIMINATION

1. Do you wash your hands at least 5 times a day? _____ _____

2. Do you brush your teeth every day? _____ _____

3. Do you shower at least every other day? _____ _____

4. Do you go to the bathroom on a regular basis? _____ _____

MENTAL FOOD

1. Do you do a good job on your homework? _____ _____

2. Do you read at home at least 3 days a week? _____ _____

3. Do you ask questions about things you want to learn more about? _____

4. Do you use good study habits to prepare for a test? _____ _____

MENTAL REST

1. Do you enjoy family vacations or outings? _____ _____

2. Do you take a break when you are stressed or frustrated? _____ _____

3. Do you look forward to "free time" and doing something just because you enjoy it? _____ _____

4. Do you practice calming down when you are stressed? _____ _____

MENTAL EXERCISE

1. Do you participate in class discussions? _____ _____

2. Do you check that homework assignments are done correctly before you turn them in? _____ _____

3. Do you like solving problems or puzzles? _____ _____

4. Do you study more than one time before taking a test or quiz? _____

MENTAL ELIMINATION

1. Do you figure out the correct answers to mistakes on tests/quizzes or papers? _____ _____

2. Do you ask questions in class when you are confused? _____ _____

3. Do you easily remember information needed for tests? _____ _____

4. Do you ask adults for help when making a difficult decision? _____ _

SPIRITUAL FOOD

1. Do you have an adult you can tell your problems to? _____ _____

2. Do you accept compliments easily? _____ _____

3. Can you name 3 or more things you are good at? _____ _____

4. Do you enjoy being with others? _____ _____

SPIRITUAL REST

1. Do you let others help you when you need something? _____ _____

2. Do you do things just to make you feel better? _____ _____

3. Do you enjoy being alone? _____ _____

4. Do you tell someone when you are afraid? _____ _____

SPIRITUAL EXERCISE

1. Do you do things for others, even before they ask for help? _____ __

2. Do you get along with your family? _____ _____

3. Do you know how to make and keep friends? _____ _____

4. Do you forgive yourself easily when you make a mistake? _____ __

SPIRITUAL ELIMINATION

1. Do you forgive others easily? _____ _____

2. Do you remain calm when you angry? _____ _____

3. Are you jealous of others if the have something or have done something

    you wish you had? _____ _____

4. Do you tell people when you are upset with them? _____ _____

MODIFIED SURVEY BAR GRAPH

PHYSICAL

1 3 5 7	8 9 10	11 12 13	14 15 16	FOOD
1 3 5 7	8 9 10	11 12 13	14 15 16	REST
1 3 5 7	8 9 10	11 12 13	14 15 16	EXERCISE
1 3 5 7	8 9 10	11 12 13	14 15 16	ELIMINATION

MENTAL

1 3 5 7	8 9 10	11 12 13	14 15 16	FOOD
1 3 5 7	8 9 10	11 12 13	14 15 16	REST
1 3 5 7	8 9 10	11 12 13	14 15 16	EXERCISE
1 3 5 7	8 9 10	11 12 13	14 15 16	ELIMINATION

SPIRITUAL

1 3 5 7	8 9 10	11 12 13	14 15 16	FOOD
1 3 5 7	8 9 10	11 12 13	14 15 16	REST
1 3 5 7	8 9 10	11 12 13	14 15 16	EXERCISE
1 3 5 7	8 9 10	11 12 13	14 15 16	ELIMINATION

MODIFIED SURVEY PIE GRAPH

MY CURRENT HEALTH PIE

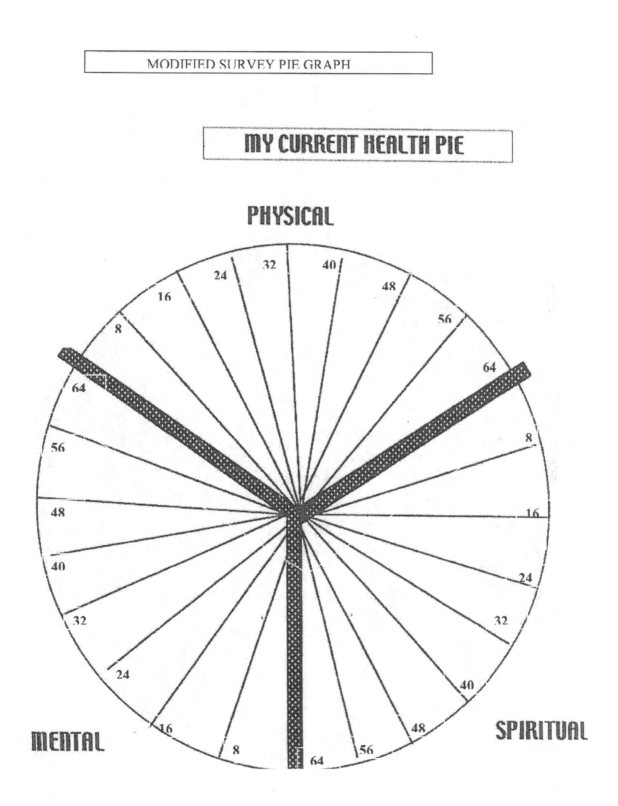

PHYSICAL

MENTAL

SPIRITUAL

GOAL SETTING GUIDELINES

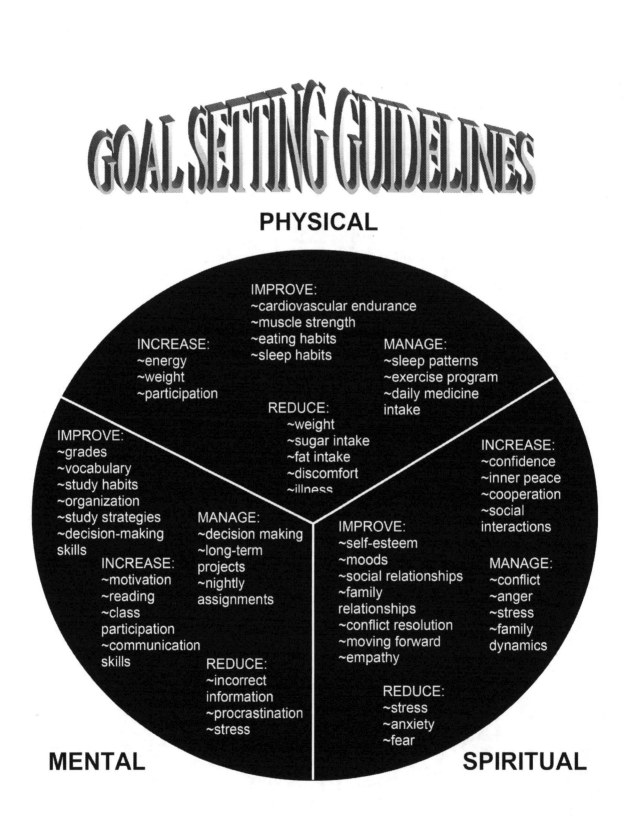

PHYSICAL

IMPROVE:
~cardiovascular endurance
~muscle strength
~eating habits
~sleep habits

INCREASE:
~energy
~weight
~participation

MANAGE:
~sleep patterns
~exercise program
~daily medicine
intake

REDUCE:
~weight
~sugar intake
~fat intake
~discomfort
~illness

IMPROVE:
~grades
~vocabulary
~study habits
~organization
~study strategies
~decision-making
skills

INCREASE:
~motivation
~reading
~class
participation
~communication
skills

MANAGE:
~decision making
~long-term
projects
~nightly
assignments

IMPROVE:
~self-esteem
~moods
~social relationships
~family
relationships
~conflict resolution
~moving forward
~empathy

INCREASE:
~confidence
~inner peace
~cooperation
~social
interactions

MANAGE:
~conflict
~anger
~stress
~family
dynamics

REDUCE:
~incorrect
information
~procrastination
~stress

REDUCE:
~stress
~anxiety
~fear

MENTAL   **SPIRITUAL**

CONTRACT FOR A HEALTHY LIFE

Name: _____ *Period:* _____

1) I wish to work on the following component of my health:

(Circle one)

Physical   Mental   Spiritual

2) I will concentrate on the daily requirement(s) of: (circle one)

Food   Exercise   Rest   Elimination

3) My goal is:

(circle one)

to improve

to manage

to increase

to reduce

4) I plan to do the following tasks or behaviors to attain my goal:

5) My strategy to evaluate and measure my progress is:

6) My "Support Person" will be: _____

Signed: _____ Date:_____

(Student's Signature)

CONTRACT FOR A HEALTHY LIFE

Support Person Agreement

Student's Name: _____

Support Person's Name: _____

Relationship to Student: _____

1. I have read the workbook and understand the definition of health and the goal of the project.

2. I understand the guidelines of a support person as one who listens, encourages, and gives advice when asked.

3. I understand that I am expected to review the measurement log and sign it weekly.

4. I understand that I am expected to complete an evaluation form at the completion of this project.

I have read the statements above and do agree to assist in this project.

Signed: _____ Date: _____

CONTRACT FOR A HEALTHY LIFE

Support Person Final Evaluation

Student's Name: _____

Support Person's Name: _____

1. Please <u>briefly</u> describe what you understood to be the student's goal and whether in your opinion he/she was successful.

2. Any suggestions for the student on how his/her project could have been more successful?

8. Please describe an attribute or strength that the student exhibited:

9. Did you enjoy your involvement in this activity? Why? Or why not?

* THANK YOU FOR YOUR TIME AND EFFORT IN SUPPORTING THIS STUDENT IN HIS/HER JOURNEY TO BALANCE HIS/HER HEALTH. PLEASE COMPLETE THIS EVALUATION FORM AND SIGN BELOW. *

Signed: _____ Date: _____

MEASUREMENT TOOLS

Selecting Your Measurement Tool

The measuring tool will enable you to objectively (numerically) and/or subjectively (observations/feelings) track your progress toward your goal. For the next six to eight weeks your recorded discoveries will specifically identify how you progress daily and weekly.

Required Data Collection:

- ✓ Day and Date
- ✓ Behavior and Actions
- ✓ Discoveries *(personal results and/or impact on others)*
- ✓ Reflection *(progress made)*

* You may create your own system to record and measure your progress, or you may choose one of the sample logs provided. *

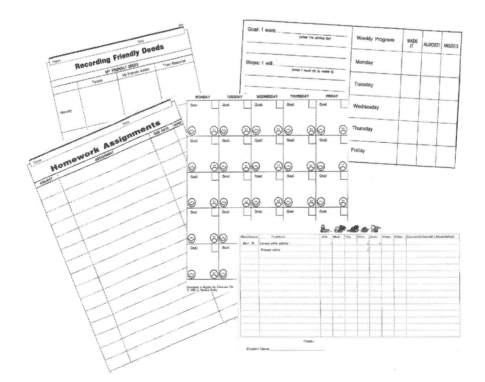

GENERAL USE

MEASUREMENT TOOLS

Weekly Contract Progress Report

*Name:*_____ *Period:* _____ *Date:* _____

1. Restate your goal for your contract project. What do you want to accomplish?

2. What are some things that have interfered with your reaching this goal?

3. Have you spoken with your support person about your progress and if so, what suggestions have been made?

4. What strategies will you use this week to ensure you are staying on task?

PHYSICAL HEALTH

<u>Measurement Tools:</u>

> - Rest & Sleep
> - Physical Exercise
> - Stress Management
> - Hygiene & Cleanliness
> - Nutrition & Eating Behavior

Habits and Behaviors

* Improve your physical fitness: strength, endurance, and/or flexibility

* Improve your hygiene: wash hands more often, and/or increase time spent brushing & flossing teeth

* Improve your diet: food choices, eating habits, and/or fluid intake

* Cut back on sugar intake

* Cut back on fat consumption

* Cut down on caffeine

* Drink 8-9 glasses of water a day

* Manage daily calories

* Sleep more at night

A Weekly Inventory of My Physical Behaviors

Student Name:_____Week of:_____

DAY	BEHAVIORS/ACTIONS	COMMENTS /DISCOVERIES

COMMENTS /DISCOVERIES
- Special circumstances
- How many times-or how long
- Time of Day/Location
- Changes you notice

F_____

_____

Sa_____

_____

Su_____

_____

M_____

_____

T_____

_____

W_____

_____

T_____

_____

A Weekly Inventory of My Eating Behaviors

Student Name: _____Week of: _____

Day Meal   Food item Comments /Discoveries.

B = Breakfast	~ Food group	~ Special circumstances
L = Lunch	~ Serving size	~ Time of day / Location
D = Dinner	~ Number of servings	~ Quality food vs. junk food
S = Snack	~ I was or wasn't hungry.	

F_____

_____

Sa_____

_____

Su_____

_____

M_____

_____

T_____

_____

W_____

_____

T_____

_____

PHYSICAL REST SLEEP LOG

| Day & Date | REST PERIODS | | SLEEP | | |
	Where? When?	How long?	Bed time	Wake up time	# Hours of sleep

MENTAL HEALTH

Measurement Tools

Improve Academic Performance

Increase Reading

Improve Vocabulary

Stress Reduction

Improve Organizational Skills

Reduce procrastination

SCHOOL
STUDY SKILLS AND HABITS

- Arrive to all classes on time

- Bring all required materials

- Participate and be attentive in class

- Take good notes

- Ask questions when confused

- Write down nightly homework and long- term assignments

- Keep locker clean and organized

- Check before leaving school that you have all materials needed

HOME
STUDY SKILLS AND HABITS

- Choose a consistent place to work that
is comfortable and well lighted

- Supply study area with materials (pens, pencils, rulers, paper, etc.)

- Before starting assignments, read directions carefully

- Check off assignments as you complete them

- Use a system to keep track of upcoming tests, long-term projects, and reports

- Proofread assignments before turning them in

- Preview and study several times before a test

READING LOG

DAY & DATE	WHERE (in class / home)	WHEN (time of day)	TITLE	START PAGE #	END PAGE#

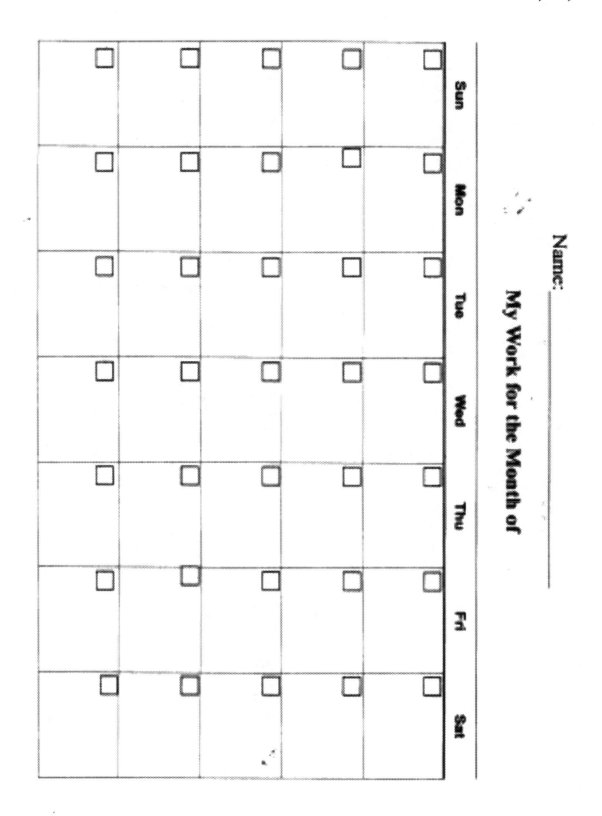

Name: _____

My Work for the Month of _____

Sun	Mon	Tue	Wed	Thu	Fri	Sat
☐	☐	☐	☐	☐	☐	☐
☐	☐	☐	☐	☐	☐	☐
☐	☐	☐	☐	☐	☐	☐
☐	☐	☐	☐	☐	☐	☐
☐	☐	☐	☐	☐	☐	☐

MY DAILY ORGANIZER

Name:_____

DATE: DATE:

                    HOME   SCHOOL   HOME   SCHOOL

AGENDA   **AGENDA**

TEXTBOOKS: **TEXTBOOKS:**

Subject: Subject:

Subject: Subject:

Subject: Subject:

Subject: Subject:

Subject: Subject:

NOTEBOOKS: **NOTEBOOKS:**

Subject: Subject:

Subject: Subject:

Subject: Subject:

Subject: Subject:

Subject: Subject:

SUPPLIES   **SUPPLIES**

Pen/pencil   Pen/pencil

Rulers   Rulers

Calculator   Calculator

Art Supplies   Art Supplies

Other: Other:

SPIRITUAL HEALTH

MEASUREMENT TOOLS

Stress Reduction

Good Deeds

Expressing Feelings

Volunteerism

SOCIAL SKILLS AND HABITS

➤ Cooperating with others

➤ Expressing your ideas or feelings

➤ Doing someone a favor

➤ Starting a conversation

➤ Leading/taking charge of a task

➤ Respecting the rights of others

➤ Saying you are sorry

➤ Ignoring someone's behavior

➤ Being polite

➤ Attentively listening to someone

➤ Settling an argument calmly

➤ Doing an act of kindness

➤ Forgiving someone

PERSONAL SKILLS AND HABITS

- Writing your feelings in a journal/diary

- Listening to or playing music

- Praying

- Meditating

- Practicing relaxation exercises

- Acknowledging your own accomplishment

- Letting someone help you

- Telling your parents about your day

- Working for a charity or a social cause

- Forgiving a mistake you made

A Weekly Inventory of My Spiritual Health Habits

Student Name:_____Week of:

Day	*Behavior/Action*	*Comments/Discoveries.*

~ *Special circumstances* ~ *Enjoyed it*
~ Time of day (AM/PM) ~ Planned to do
~ How long/how much? ~ Did it without thinking
~ At school/home/other   ~ Was asked to do it
~ Feel less stresses_____ ~ Better mood

F_____

_____

Sa_____

_____

Su_____

_____

M_____

_____

T_____

_____

W_____

_____

T_____

_____

A Weekly Inventory of My Spiritual Health Behaviors

Student Name:_____Week of:

Behavior	Frequency	Day of Week	Location	Impact
	(X= Each time it happened)	(M-T-W-R-F- Sat.-Sun)	S=School H= Home O= Other	How you felt - How others felt and/or responded to you
Felt good about an accomplishment				
Asked for help				
Reflected in a journal				
Told someone your feelings				
Listened to/played music				
Prayed/meditated/yoga				
Told parents about my day				
Forgave someone				
Settled an argument calmly				
Apologized to someone				
Did an act of kindness				
Gave a compliment				
Worked for a charity/cause				

Week	Sunday		Monday		Tuesday		Wednesday		Thursday		Friday		Saturday		Total	
	Nice to Brother	Help Around House	Nice to Brother	Help Around House	Nice to Brother	Help Around House	Nice to Brother	Help Around House	Nice to Brother	Help Around House	Nice to Brother	Help Around House	Nice to Brother	Help Around House	Nice to Brother	Help Around House
1																
2																
3																
4																
5																
6																

Student Name: _____

Contract for a Healthy Life

"Putting It All Together"
FINAL PACKET

Visual Presentation Guide
Oral Presentation Guide

Project Rubric
Support Person Evaluation Form

DUE DATE:

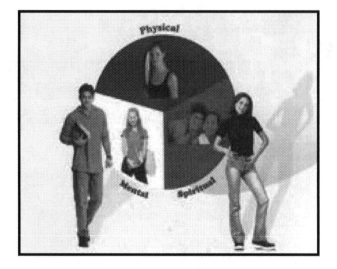

_____Step 1: Retake your Wellness Survey.

_____Step 2: Complete 2nd column of "My Wellness Survey Results" page (*analyzing pre-post results*).

_____Step 3: Complete the 2nd pie and bar graphs using new results and same color scheme.

_____Step 4: Ask support person to complete evaluation sheet.

_____Step 5: Answer the personal reflection questions.

_____Step 6: Attach at least one sample measuring tool.

_____Step 7: Create a cover page with title, student name and period

_____Step 8: Staple together the following (in this order):

> ➤ Cover page
>
> ➤ My Wellness Survey Results worksheet
>
> ➤ Graphs: Before and after graphs
>
> ➤ Answers to the reflection questions
>
> ➤ Signed & completed Support Person Evaluation
>
> ➤ Sample measuring tool(s)
>
> ➤ Grading Sheet with student column completed

	ABOVE EXPECTATION	MEETS EXPECTATION	BELOW EXPECTATION	Student	Teacher
Project Content: "Putting it all together" 0-10 POINTS	Has beyond all the requires elements - Decorative/creative Cover Page - Pre-post bar and pie graphs (4) with proper color coding - My Wellness Survey Results worksheet (both columns completed) - Personal Reflection Questions - Signed & completes Support Person Evaluation - Sample Measuring Tools (2 or more) - Completed student column of grading sheet 10 POINTS	Has the requires elements - Cover Page - Pre-post bar or pie graphs (2) - Survey results worksheet - Personal Reflection Questions - Support Person Evaluation - Sample Measuring Tool - Grading sheet 8 POINTS	Lacks 2 or more of the following requirements: - Cover Page - Pre-post bar or pie graphs - Survey results worksheet - Personal Reflection Questions - Support Person Evaluation - Sample Measuring Tool - Grading sheet 6-0 POINTS		
Personal Reflection Questions	Format: Complete full sentence answers with a minimum of 3 sentences per question. Content: Demonstrates an ability to reflect and assess own level of wellness. Demonstrates a strong understanding of balancing one's physical, mental and spiritual health, daily requirements and goal setting. Demonstrates conviction and desire to make healthful choices. 80-72 POINTS	Format: Complete full sentence answers with a minimum of 2 sentences per question. Content: Demonstrates a good understanding of personal project's connection to wellness, the balancing of one's health and goal setting. 72 - 56 POINTS	Format: Incomplete sentences and/ or less than 2 sentences per question. Content: Insufficient or inaccurate connections of personal project to wellness, the balancing of one's health and goal setting. 55-0 POINTS		

| Format and Effort

0-10 POINTS | Shows excellent organization, effort and preparation.
- On time
-Has minimal grammar and spelling
-Neat, easy to read and/or has extra elements
-All pages fastened together and in order
-Completed student column of grading sheet

10 – 8 POINTS | Shows a good degree of effort and preparation.
- On time
- Shows a degree of proof reading and organization
- Neat and easy to read
- Pages stapled together in order

7-6 POINTS | Shows minimal effort in preparation or presentation of final product.

- Turned in late
-Shows little to no evidence of proof reading and organization
- Messy and/or difficult to read

5-0 POINTS | | |

CONTRACT FOR A HEALTHY LIFE PROJECT GRADING SHEET

Student's Name: _____

Per: _____

Score= _____   Final Grade=_____

Contract for a Healthy Life

FINAL PROJECT GUIDELINES

Your presentation must demonstrate your understanding of the definition of health and the 4 daily requirements needed to nurture and balance each area of health. You will identify how you assessed your wellness before, during, and after your eight week program.

Your final grade will be based on a visual and oral presentation.

YOUR POSTER <u>MUST</u> CONTAIN:

1. A "before" and "after" pie or bar graph
2. A brief summary including:
    - ✓ Your rationale (why you chose the area of health and your specific goal)
    - ✓ Your strategy and measurement tools (how you planned to improve and how you measured your progress)
    - ✓ Statement accessing your success and what progress was achieved
    - ✓ A sample of your measuring tool (log)

Improving my Physical Health

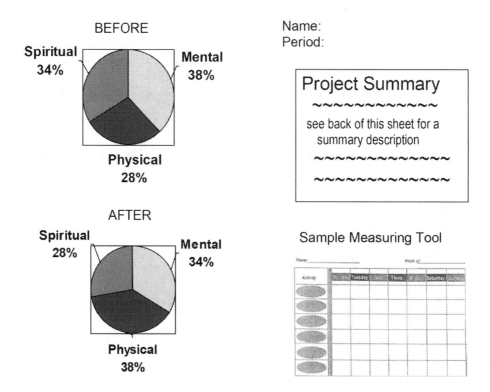

YOUR PROJECT SUMMARY <u>MUST</u> CONTAIN:

✓ Your Rationale:

- What area of health, daily requirement(s) did you select to work on?

- Which survey results lead you to choose that area of health?

- What was your specific goal?

- Why did you choose this goal?

****<u>Hint:</u> Refer to your contract form and survey worksheet*

✓ Your Strategy and Measurement Tools:

- What specific tasks or behaviors did you target?

- Did you want to improve, add or reduce these behaviors?

- How did you measure your short-term and long-term progress and achievements?

** *<u>Hint:</u> Refer to your contract form and your measuring tool.*

✓ Your Progress and Accomplishments:

- • Were there any setbacks or changes along the way?

- • Did your post-survey results indicate improvement in the desired area of health?

- • Did your post-survey show improvement in any of the other areas of health?

- • In what ways have you noticed improvement or changes?

- • Did anyone else (family, friends, teachers) notice any changes?

- • What was your greatest accomplishment?

** <u>*Hint:*</u> *Refer to your measuring tool, post-survey worksheets and graphs, your update worksheet, and your support person evaluation. Also, ask your support person for their thoughts.*

VISUAL PRESENTATION GUIDE

Reflection Questions

1. Did you identify the health area that you targeted for improvement?

2. Did you clearly explain what your goal was?

3. Did you clearly label and explain the before and after pie graphs?

4. Did you include an example or explanation of your short-term strategies and measurement tool(s)?

5. Are your visuals informative and easy to understand?

6. Is your text informative and well written?

7. Is your poster neat and logically organized?

8. Is your poster attractive to the audience?

9. Did you use any new and interesting ideas to create your poster?

10. Was your poster turned in on time?

ORAL PRESENTATION GUIDE

YOUR ORAL PRESENTATION MUST CONTAIN:

1. Complete and prepared answers to the reflection questions

2. Description and explanation of your visual poster

3. Explanation of your rationale, goals, progress, and results

Reflection Questions

1. What area of Health did I chose for my Contract and why?

2. Which daily requirements did I concentrate on? Why?

3. Which specific behaviors did I target and why did I choose them?
   *** Describe your measuring tool on your poster***

4. Did I achieve any overall improvement to my health?
   *** Explain any changes in your before and after graphs***

5. What benefits did I experience? Was I successful? Did others notice any changes? (If not, what changes might have helped me be more successful?)

6. How did I utilize my support person? Was the person helpful? Why or why not? Did this project change our relationship?

7. What did I like the most about this project?

8. What was the hardest part of this project?

9. What have I learned from this project? Has this project had any lasting effect on me?

10. How will this experience be helpful in my future?

(Your reflection should include how the process of recognizing the need for change and altering a behavior can improve many areas of your health, not just the area you focused on for this project.)

ASSESSMENTS

CONTRACT FOR A HEALTHY LIFE

Support Person Final Evaluation

Student's Name: _____

Support Person's Name: _____

1. Please <u>briefly</u> describe what you understood to be the student's goal, and whether in your opinion he/she was successful?

2. Any suggestions for the student on how his/her project could have been more successful?

3. Please describe an attribute or strength that the student exhibited:

4. Did you enjoy your involvement in this activity? Why? Or why not?

*I thank you for supporting this student on his/her beginning journey to a better balanced life of health and wellness. * Please sign below. *

Signed: _____ **Date:** _____

Rubric:	Poster Content *(0-50 pts)*	Poster Design & Visual Appeal (0-10pts)	Oral Presentation Content (0-30 pts)	Oral Presentation Delivery (0-10 pts)
Awesome	**Project Summary:** ___Clearly connects survey results to the area of health selected and rationale for choosing it. ___Identifies specific behavioral goal(s) that were targeted. ___Describes plan or strategy used and method to track progress. ___Offers references to post survey and measuring tool to demonstrate changes that progress, pitfalls and/or successes. **Visuals:** ___Sample measuring tool included and described. ___Contains well labeled before and after pie graphs	___Easy to read and very neat. ___Poster's layout is logical and shows good effort. ___Title is descriptive and informative. ___Use of unique design and/or text. ___Pleasing use of graphics, colors and/or artwork.	___Clearly explained goal and rationale for desired change. ___Described selected behaviors and strategies used as methods to reach goal. ___Identified support person's role and effectiveness. ___Shared thoughtful reflection about progress, pitfalls and successes. ___Shared personal impact or affect this project may have on future.	___Demonstrated preparation and forethought. ___Thoroughly explained poster and its visuals. ___Showed a positive, serious and confident attitude. ___Used a loud and clear voice.
Acceptable	**Project Summary:** ___Explains area of health selected and reason for choosing it. ___Identifies goal that was targeted. ___Describes method of tracking progress. ___Identifies progress, pitfalls, and/or successes experienced. **Visuals:** ___Sample measuring tool included. ___Presents before and after pie graphs.	___Mostly neat. ___Shows effort. ___Fairly logical layout. ___Has a title. ___Text is readable. ___Some use of color and artwork.	___Identified area of health targeted, desired change and the goal selected. ___Described behaviors and explained measuring tool used. ___Identified support person and why he/she was chosen. ___Explains progress achieved and whether will continue working on goal.	___Demonstrated some preparation. ___Explained poster and its visuals. ___Showed a serious attitude. ___Audience could hear presentation.
Unacceptable	___Lacks two or more of the following: project description, pie graphs or sample measurement tool.	___Somewhat disorganized ___Difficult to read ___Elements used are irrelevant or distract from appearance.	___Missing discussion of several required contract elements. ___Does not include insight or reflection regarding this project.	___No sign of preparation. ___Attitude lacked seriousness and effort.

CONTRACT FOR A HEALTHY LIFE PROJECT

Grading Sheet

Student Name:_____ **Per.** _____

	Possible Points	*Points Earned*
Poster Content	**(0-50 points)**	_____
Poster Design & Appeal	**(0-10 points)**	_____
Oral Content	**(0-30 points)**	_____
Oral Delivery	**(0-10 points)**	_____

TOTAL POINTS EARNED =   _____

FINAL GRADE:

COMMENTS:

Student Name: _____ Period 1

	Content of Presentation	Poster Design	Visual Appeal of Poster
AWESOME	~ Detailed project summary ~ Area of concentration clearly identified ~ Complete description and explanation of strategy and progress. ~ Detailed explanation of the before and after pie graphs ~ Shows and explains measurement tool. ~ Discuss role and effectiveness of support person **(70 points)**	~ Title is descriptive and informative ~ Easy to read text. ~ Neat. ~ Logical layout. **(10 points)**	~ Use of unique design and/or text. ~ Pleasing use of graphics, artwork and colors to have poster stand out.
ACCEPTABLE	~ Brief project description ~ Generally identify the area of concentration. ~ Presents both before and after graphs ~ Presents measurement tool used **(60 points)**	~ Has a title. ~ Readable text. ~ Mostly neat. ~ Fairly logical layout. **(8 points)**	~ Use of some unique elements. ~ Good use of color.
UNACCEPTABLE	~ Lacks two or more required content: project description, graphs or measurement tools. **(50 points)**	~ Somewhat disorganized ~ Difficult to read text. ~ Elements used distract from appearance and make hard to read. **(3 points)**	~ Use of little color. ~ Little evidence of effort or creativity. **(10 points)**

Total Points= _____ Grade: ____

GIVE THE GIFT OF

CONTRACT FOR a HEALTHY LIFE

to Friends, Family, and Colleagues
Check Your Leading Bookstore or Order Here

Yes, I want _____ copies of Contract for a Healthy Life at $____
each plus $_____ shipping per book (Connecticut residents please add
$_____ sales tax per book). Allow up to 15 days for delivery.

Yes, I am interested in having the author speak or give a seminar to my
company, association, school, or organization. Please send information.

My check or money order for $_____ is enclosed.
Please charge my: ☐ Visa   ☐ MasterCard
                  ☐ Discover   ☐ American Express

Name_____

Organization_____

Address_____

City/State/Zip_____

Phone_____E-Mail_____

Card#_____

Exp. Date_____Signature_____

Please make your check payable and return to
Author House Publishers
Address
Call your credit card order to: phone #
Or fax to #
Or order online at www.authorhouse.com

About the Author

Cathleen Hamill is a health educator with the Fairfield Connecticut school system. She began her career teaching physical education and coaching at the high school level. For 13 years she has been teaching middle school health to 6th, 7th, and 8th grade students at Fairfield Woods Middle School. Cathleen lives in Connecticut and continues to teach at Fairfield Woods Middle School in Fairfield, Ct. She has initiated numerous creative health projects that encourage hands-on learning for students. Contract for A Healthy Life is taught as part of the middle school health program. It's also used in various school districts to implement behavior modification for high-risk youths. Cathleen also teaches Bibliotherapy Health; a teaching style that offers stories whose characters are coping with a health issue.